T0200119

Practical management of the pregnant patient with rheumatic disease

Practical management of the pregnant patient with rheumatic disease

Edited by

KAREN SCHREIBER, MD

Danish Hospital for Rheumatic Diseases, Sonderborg, Denmark

ELIZA CHAKRAVARTY, MD

Arthritis and Clinical Immunology, Oklahoma Medical Research Foundation, USA

MONIKA ØSTENSEN, MD, PhD

Department of Rheumatology, Sorlandet Hospital, Kristiansand, Norway

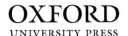

OXFORD
UNIVERSITY PRESS

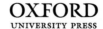

OXFORD
UNIVERSITY PRESS

Great Clarendon Street, Oxford, OX2 6DP,
United Kingdom

Oxford University Press is a department of the University of Oxford.
It furthers the University's objective of excellence in research, scholarship,
and education by publishing worldwide. Oxford is a registered trade mark of
Oxford University Press in the UK and in certain other countries

© Oxford University Press 2021

The moral rights of the authors have been asserted

First Edition published in 2021

Impression: 1

Published in the United States of America by Oxford University Press
198 Madison Avenue, New York, NY 10016, United States of America

British Library Cataloguing in Publication Data

Data available

Library of Congress Control Number: 2020936530

ISBN 978–0–19–884509–6

DOI: 10.1093/med/9780198845096.001.0001

Printed and bound by
CPI Group (UK) Ltd, Croydon, CR0 4YY

Foreword

When I was a first-year medical student the first deaths I witnessed were those of a pregnant woman with systemic lupus erythematosus (SLE) and her stillborn child. The experience was memorable both because of the deaths and because, at a Morbidity & Mortality Conference a few weeks later, I saw expert physicians, at one of the most famous hospitals in the United States, fail to offer an explanation. "It happens," they said, and shrugged their shoulders. "Pregnancy and lupus are a lethal combination." Medical certainty about this point was great. More than a decade before the Supreme Court decision *Roe v Wade* legalized abortion in the United States a diagnosis of SLE was an acceptable reason for elective termination.

Not all patients, of course, agreed. Some chose to continue their pregnancies. When they did, contemporary *ideés reçues* required pre-emptive, aggressive immunosuppression for all patients, well or ill. There was a basis for the recommendation: Pregnant SLE patients' maternal mortality rates were 34 times higher, and fetal mortality rates 4 times higher, than the rates of women who did not have SLE.[1]

By the 1970s informed, assertive patients questioned the advice that they accept either termination or pre-emptive immunosuppression. Physicians in Mexico, Norway, England, France, Sweden, the United States, Italy, Spain, Israel, Holland, and many other countries re-examined the details of rheumatic disease pregnancies. They learned to distinguish between SLE and non-SLE pregnancy complications; identify clinical predictors of maternal and fetal risk; recognize and understand antiphospholipid and anti-Ro/La antibodies; personalize treatment recommendations and offer prophylaxis for the mothers and fetuses at risk.

In 1992 Michael Yaron called together, in Jerusalem, the *First International Conference on Rheumatic Diseases in Pregnancy* (its 11th iteration is scheduled to take place in 2021, under the leadership of authors of this book.) The Conference encouraged specialty clinics throughout the world to share experiences with pregnant rheumatic disease patients and to propose new management guidelines. The impact of this and subsequent Conferences was dramatic. By the mid-2010s maternal and fetal deaths fell to 5 and 3 times those of non-SLE patients, 10-fold and 2-fold decreases—not yet satisfactory but far better than before.[2]

To what to attribute the improvement? Not to new medications or paradigm-shifted understanding of either SLE or of pregnancy. The improvement is attributable to more widely applied, careful, individualized attention to detail and intelligent, tailored, focused care—in other words, to the details of management more than to advances of

---

[1] Mehta B, Luo Y, Xu J, Sammaritano L, Salmon J, Lockshin M, Goodman S, Ibrahim S. Trends in maternal and fetal outcomes among pregnant women with systemic lupus erythematosus in the United States. Ann Intern Med 2019; doi:10.7326/M19-0120

[2] Buyon JP, Yaron M, Lockshin M D. First international conference on rheumatic diseases in pregnancy. Arthritis Rheum 1993 Jan;36(1):59-64. doi: 10.1002/art.1780360110. PMID: 8424837 DOI: 10.1002/art.1780360110

science, exemplary care that can and now should be available to all pregnant rheumatic disease patients.

The pages of this book offer the instructions in contemporary, easy to read, and pragmatic management rules for physicians and their patients. Individual chapters guide physicians in the prevention and treatment of thromboses, pulmonary arterial hypertension, renal disease, antibodies, lactation, medications, infections, vaccinations, flares, rare diseases, and many other rheumatic and non-rheumatic disease pregnancy complications. Although front-line physicians may not often encounter pregnant rheumatic disease patients, when they need information they will find today's best management practices in this book. They and their patients can learn to anticipate complications, precisely target treatment, and choose or decline aggressive anti-rheumatic disease therapy according to need.

Decades ago I, the first-year medical student, was told that our patients' prognoses were invariably dire. That is no longer true. Pregnancies are now reasonably safe and feasible for most rheumatic disease patients. Physicians who follow the guidelines outlined in this book can look forward to healthy outcomes for both mother and child.

Michael D. Lockshin, MD, MACR
Director, Barbara Volcker Center for Women
and Rheumatic Diseases
Hospital for Special Surgery
Professor of Medicine and Obstetrics-Gynecology
Weill Cornell Medicine
New York, NY, USA

Preface

Many women with rheumatic diseases are of childbearing age and many have not completed their families before disease onset. With increasingly improved control of autoimmune and inflammatory disease, the physical burden of childbearing and childrearing has lessened, and more women with these conditions wish to become pregnant. It is essential that specialists from different medical specialties, midwives, and nurses gain familiarity with the pregnancy, antenatal care, and care in the post-partum period. A growing body of literature studies all clinical and immunological aspects of reproductive health issues in women with chronic autoimmune diseases. However, the increasing amount of data can make real-time decision making cumbersome without a thorough review of the literature or more comprehensive textbooks. With increasing data regarding the role of underlying disease activity on pregnancy outcomes and updated information regarding risk stratification of medication use in pregnancy, providers must have easy access to summary recommendations for management of pregnant women with autoimmune diseases whenever they require health care.

This book will bring these data to the clinician in a distilled and clinically relevant manner that can be easily applied to the varying situations that may occur in the clinical setting, with references to more detailed background and primary studies for those who desire a more in-depth review of the material.

This book is intended as a quick-access guide of the most up-to-date understanding of the interplay between pregnancy and rheumatic diseases and principles of management before, during and after pregnancy assisting in decision making regarding treatment of women with autoimmune diseases. This collection of 70 cases covers pregnancy counselling, the management of disease flares, thromboembolic disease, the management of patients with end organ disease, advice on medications, obstetric complications, infections and the management of rare diseases in women with rheumatic diseases before and during pregnancy and postpartum. We intend to provide concise recommendations for all providers who may encounter women of childbearing age including rheumatologists, gynaecologists, paediatricians, primary care providers, and health professionals dealing with pre-conceptional and pregnant women with rheumatic diseases.

We are indebted and grateful to all our co-authors, who have provided excellent contributions within their field of expertise.

The editors

Acknowledgement

We acknowledge Renata Donciu for her artistic contribution.

Karen Schreiber
Eliza Chakravarty
Monika Østensen

Contents

Contributors

Maria Rhona G. Bergantin, Department of Rheumatology, University of Santo Tomas, Faculty of Medicine & Surgery, Manila, Philippines

Bonnie L. Bermas, Internal Medicine, UT Southwestern Medical Center, Dallas, USA

Hannah Blakey, Department of Renal Medicine, Queen Elizabeth Hospital Birmingham, Birmingham, UK

Kate Bramham, Women and Children's Health, King's College London, London, UK

D. Ware Branch, Maternal-Fetal Medicine, University of Utah Medical Center, Salt Lake City, USA

Eliza Chakravarty, Arthritis and Clinical Immunology, Oklahoma Medical Research Foundation, Oklahoma City, USA

Megan Clowse, Department of Medicine, Duke University School of Medicine, Durham, USA

Andrew James Doyle, Thrombosis and Haemophilia, Guy's and St Thomas' NHS Foundation Trust, London, UK

Ian Giles, Centre for Rheumatology, University College London, London, UK

Jon Golenbiewski, Division of Rheumatology, Department of Medicine, Duke University School of Medicine, Durham, USA

Beverley Jane Hunt, Thrombosis and Haemophilia, Guy's and St Thomas' NHS Foundation Trust, London, UK

David Isenberg, Centre for Rheumatology, University College London, London, UK

Søren Jacobsen, Copenhagen Lupus and Vasculitis Clinic, Center for Rheumatology and Spine Diseases, Copenhagen University Hospital, Rigshospitalet, Copenhagen, Denmark

Sandra V. Navarra, Department of Rheumatology, University of Santo Tomas, Manila, Philippines

Fionnuala Ní Ainle, Department of Haematology, Mater Misericordiae University Hospital, Dublin, Ireland

Roseann O'Doherty, Department of Haematology, Mater Misericordiae University Hospital, Dublin, Ireland

Monika Østensen, Department of Rheumatology, Sorlandet Hospital, Kristiansand, Norway

Massimo Radin, Center of Research of Immunopathology and Rare Diseases-Coordinating Center of Piemonte and Valle d'Aosta Network for Rare Diseases, Department of Clinical and Biological Sciences, and SCDU Nephrology and Dialysis, S. Giovanni Bosco Hospital, Turin, Italy

Christof Schaefer, Charité Pharmakovigilanzzentrum Embryonaltoxikologie, Charité Universitätsmedizin, Berlin, Germany

Karen Schreiber, Danish Hospital for Rheumatic Diseases, Sonderborg, Denmark; Copenhagen Lupus and Vasculitis Clinic, Rigshospitalet, Copenhagen, Denmark and Thrombosis and Haemophilia, Guy's and St Thomas' NHS Foundation Trust, London, UK

Savino Sciascia, Center of Research of Immunopathology and Rare Diseases-Coordinating Center of Piemonte and Valle d'Aosta Network for Rare Diseases, Department of Clinical and Biological Sciences, and SCDU Nephrology and Dialysis, S. Giovanni Bosco Hospital, Turin, Italy

Muhammad Shipa, North Middlesex University Hospital NHS Trust, UK

Cara D. Varley, Oregon Health and Science University School of Medicine, Portland, USA

Kevin L. Winthrop, Center for Infectious Disease Studies, Oregon Health and Science University, Portland, USA

Abbreviations

6MP	6-mercaptopurine
AAV	ANCA-associated vasculitis
ACEi	angiotensin-converting enzyme inhibitors
ACIP	Advisory Committee on Immunization Practices
aCL	anticardiolipin
ACOG	American College of Obstetricians and Gynecologists
ACPA	anti-citrullinated peptide antibodies
ACR	albumin–creatinine ratio
AFI	amniotic fluid volume as an index
AKI	acute kidney injury
ALT	alanine aminotransferase
AMH	anti-Müllerian hormone
ANA	antinuclear antibody
ANCA	antineutrophil cytoplasmic antibody
AOSD	adult onset Still's disease
aPL	antiphospholipid antibodies
APS	antiphospholipid syndrome
ARB	angiotensin receptor blockers
ART	assisted reproduction technique
AS	ankylosing spondylitis
ASDAS	ankylosing spondylitis disease activity score
ASH	American Society of Hematology
aSS	anti-synthetase antibody
AST	aspartate aminotransferase
AV	atrioventricular
axSpA	axial spondyloarthritis
AZA	azathioprine
BAL	bronchoalveolar lavage
BCG	Bacille–Calmette Guérin
BD	Behçet's disease
BMI	body mass index
BP	blood pressure
BPP	biophysical profile test
BSR	British Society for Rheumatology
C3/C4	complement protein 3 and 4
CAPS	catastrophic APS
CBC	complete blood count
CCHB	congenital complete heart block
CHB	congenital heart block
CHIPS	Control of Hypertension In Pregnancy Study

CK	creatine kinase
CKD	chronic kidney disease
CNS	central nervous system
COX	cyclooxygenase
CRP	C-reactive protein
CS	Caesarean section
CSF	cerebrospinal fluid
CT	computed tomography
CTD-PAH	connective tissue disease-associated PAH
CTG	cardiotocography
CTPA	computed tomography pulmonary angiography
CUS	compression ultrasound
CYC	cyclophosphamide
CYP	cytochrome
CZP	certolizumab pegol
DAH	diffuse alveolar haemorrhage
DAS	disease activation score
dcSSc	diffuse cutaneous systemic sclerosis
DiPEP	Diagnosis of PE in Pregnancy
DLCO	diffusion capacity
DLE	discoid lupus erythematosus
DM	dermatomyositis
DMARD	disease-modifying antirheumatic drug
DNA	deoxyribonucleic acid
DOAC	direct oral anticoagulants
DRVVT	dilute Russell's viper venom time
dsDNA	double-stranded DNA
DVT	deep vein thrombosis
ECG	electrocardiogram
echo	echocardiogram
eGFR	estimated glomerular filtration rate
EGPA	eosinophilic granulomatosis with polyangiitis
ELISA	enzyme-linked immunosorbent assay
EMA	European Medicines Agency
ENA	extractable nuclear antigens
ESR	erythrocyte sedimentation rate
ESRD	end stage renal disease
EU	European Union
EULAR	European League against Rheumatism
FDA	Federal Drug Administration
FVC	forced vital capacity
GAPSS	Global Antiphospholipid Score
GDM	gestational diabetes
GFR	glomerular filtration rate
GPA	granulomatosis with polyangiitis

GPL	IgG phospholipid (1 GPL unit is 1 microgram of IgG antibody)
HAV	hepatitis A virus
HBSAg	hepatitis B surface antigen
HBV	hepatitis B virus
hCG	human chorionic gonadotropin
HCQ	hydroxychloroquine
HCV	hepatitis C virus
HCVRNA	hepatitis C virus ribonucleic acid
HD	hypertensive disorder
HELLP	haemolysis, elevated liver enzymes, and a low platelet count
HEV	hepatitis E virus
HG	hyperemesis gravidarum
HIT	heparin-induced thrombocytopenia
HIV	human immunodeficiency virus
HPV	human papillomavirus
HRCT	high resolution computed tomography
IBD	inflammatory bowel disease
ICU	intensive care unit
IGA	immunoglobulin A
IgG	immunoglobulin G
IGRA	interferon-gamma release assay
IIM	inflammatory myopathies
ILD	interstitial lung disease
INR	international normalized ratio
ISTH	International Society for Thrombosis and Haemostasis
ITP	idiopathic thrombocytopenic purpura
IUD	intrauterine device
IUGR	intrauterine growth restriction
IV	intravenous
IVF	in vitro fertilization
IVIG	intravenous immunoglobulin
JDM	juvenile dermatomyositis
LA	lupus anticoagulant
LDA	low-dose aspirin
LDL-C	low-density lipoprotein cholesterol
LEF	leflunomide
LMP	last menstrual period
LMWH	low-molecular-weight heparin
LUF	luteinized unruptured follicle syndrome
MCP	metacarpophalangeal
MCTD	mixed connective tissue disease
MMF	mycophenolate mofetil
MMR	measles, mumps, rubella
MPL	IgM phospholipid (1 MPL unit is 1 microgram of IgM antibody)
MR	magnetic resonance

MRI	magnetic resonance imaging
MTX	methotrexate
NICE	National Institute for Health and Care Excellence
NSAID	non-steroidal anti-inflammatory drug
NSR	normal sinus rhythm
NST	non-stress test
OCs	oral contraceptives
OR	odds ratio
$PaCO_2$	partial pressure of arterial carbon dioxide
PA-DVT	pregnancy-associated DVT
PAH	pulmonary arterial hypertension
PA-VTE	pregnancy-associated VTE
PCR	protein–creatinine ratio
PD	pharmacodynamic
PE	pulmonary embolism
PET	pre-eclampsia toxaemia
PEX	plasma exchange
PGA	Physician's Global Assessment
PIP	proximal interphalangeal
PK	pharmacokinetic
PlGF	placental growth factor
PM	polymyositis
PPH	postpartum haemorrhage
PPROM	preterm premature rupture of membranes
PROM	premature rupture of membranes
PsA	psoriatic arthritis
PTB	pre-term birth
RA	rheumatoid arthritis
RCOG	Royal College of Obstetricians and Gynaecologists
RCT	randomized controlled trial
RILD	rapidly progressive interstitial lung disease
RR	relative risk
RTX	rituximab
SCLE	subacute cutaneous lupus erythematosus
sFlt-1	soluble Fms-like tyrosine kinase receptor-1
SGA	small-for-gestational-age
SLE	systemic lupus erythematosus
SLEPDAI	Systemic Lupus Erythematosus Pregnancy Disease Activity Index
SmPC	summary of product characteristics
SRC	scleroderma renal crisis
SS	Sjögren syndrome
SSA or anti-SSA	anti-Sjögren's-syndrome-related antigen A (also called anti-Ro)
SSB or anti-SSB	anti-Sjögren's-syndrome-related antigen B (also called anti-La)
SSc	systemic sclerosis
SZ	sulfasalazine

T2T	treat-to-target
TAK	Takayasu arteritis
TB	tuberculosis
Tdap	tetanus toxoid, reduced diphtheria toxoid, and acellular pertussis
TIA	transient ischaemic attack
TMA	thrombotic microangiopathy
TNF	tumour necrosis factor
TNFi	TNF inhibitor
TPMT	thiopurine S-methyltransferase
TSVT	Taipan snake venom time
U1RNP	U1-ribonucleoprotein
UCTD	undifferentiated connective tissue disease
UFH	unfractionated heparin
US	ultrasonography
V/Q scan	ventilation/perfusion lung scan
VEGF	vascular endothelial growth factor
VKA	vitamin K antagonists
VTE	venous thromboembolism
vWF	von Willebrand factor
VZIg	varicella-zoster immunoglobulin
VZV	varicella-zoster virus
WHO	World Health Organization

SECTION I
COUNSELLING

1
Important points of
pre-pregnancy counselling

Monika Østensen

Introduction

Rheumatic and autoimmune diseases have a preference for the female gender and occur frequently in women of childbearing age. Substantial progress made in diagnosis and therapy has made it possible for many women with rheumatic diseases (RD) to have children. However, a successful outcome of pregnancy requires planning and finding the right time for pregnancy with the best prospect for maternal and child health. Predictors contributing to maternal and child outcomes are shown in Table 1.1.

The task of health care providers (HCP) is to assist women with RD in making the right decisions about timing of pregnancy, management, and monitoring during pregnancy. The prerequisite for doing so is to address family planning in each patient of fertile years early on and regularly under follow-up. The initiative for counselling must come from the clinician since patients most at need for pre-pregnancy counselling may not address family planning spontaneously and miss important information. The patient's life plan and her fertility goals are the starting point for the discussion. Evaluation of the severity of disease in the individual patient, stage of disease, and predictors of future development form the background for the discussion of reproduction issues (1).

Several surveys have shown that 30–60% of patients of childbearing age are not offered counselling on family planning (2). The failure to address family planning on a regular basis in all patients of fertile years increases the risk of unplanned or ill-timed pregnancy, for example at stages of active disease or while on embryotoxic/foetotoxic drugs. Knowledge about a patient's family planning can guide the selection of immunosuppressive therapy by giving preference to pregnancy-compatible and fast-acting drugs. Follow-up visits may be intensified because a patient plans a first-time pregnancy at an age of >35 years.

Counselling should be guided by the questions and concerns the patient has regarding pregnancy and raising children. The aim is to empower the patient to make informed decisions in and around pregnancy (3). In the encounter, the HCP needs to learn what the patient already knows, which information she has got from other HCP, from family, friends, other patients, or from the internet. A primary goal of counselling is eliminating unfounded anxieties and to give balanced information regarding possible maternal and foetal risks arising either from the disease or from therapy. Psychological skill is needed when informing about risks such as congenital heart

Table 1.1 Predictors of pregnancy outcome

Positive pregnancy outcome	Adverse pregnancy outcome
Planned pregnancy	Unplanned pregnancy
Disease in remission	Disease active at conception
No or few comorbidities, no organ damage present	Comorbidities and/or organ damage present
Patient on stable pregnancy-compatible medication	Frequent change of therapy or stop of all medications prior to conception
Patient well informed and partaking in decisions	Lack of pre-conception counselling and confusion by contradictory advice
Coordinated interdisciplinary care during pregnancy	Lack of communication between HCPs

block (CHB). A positive attitude is reassuring for the patient. Points to consider for structuring the conversation are given in Table 1.2.

Not all women with RD face high-risk pregnancies. As shown in Table 1.3 there are great differences between RDs regarding the disease course during pregnancy and pregnancy outcome. The general trend is further modified by the stage of disease, disease activity at conception, the extent and location of organ involvement, presence of autoantibodies, comorbidities, and treatment with drugs. A woman with arthritis in a few joints, with no autoantibodies, and no organ involvement, or comorbidities does not face more risks in pregnancy than a non-diseased woman. By contrast, patients with extensive polyarticular arthritis, with inflammation, or damage in internal organs, with comorbidities, or autoantibodies that affect pregnancy may experience severe complications during pregnancy. These include pregnancy loss, hypertension in pregnancy, gestational diabetes, pre-eclampsia, and pre-term delivery. Adverse child outcomes like intrauterine growth restriction, pre-term delivery, low birth weight, and perinatal morbidity, and mortality are also increased in mothers with active, uncontrolled disease. This underlines the importance of entering pregnancy in a stage of low disease activity or remission regardless of diagnosis. Well-controlled maternal disease is the most important condition to secure an uncomplicated pregnancy and a healthy child.

Individual factors like education, socio-economic status, lifestyle, and access to health care are equally of importance. Points for risk assessment and stratification of risk are given in Table 1.4. High-risk pregnancies require coordinated interdisciplinary monitoring and management throughout pregnancy. Low-risk and many moderate-risk pregnancies can be supervised by the rheumatologist/specialist in internal medicine in collaboration with the primary physician, the obstetrician, and associated HCP.

Some patients have risk factors that suggest postponing pregnancy or to discourage pregnancy altogether. Very active disease, acute inflammation in a vital organ, recent thrombosis, or therapy with a teratogenic drug are reasons to postpone pregnancy.

Table 1.2 Counselling adapted to reproduction stages

Stage	Patient concerns	Points for counselling
	Not interested to have a pregnancy now or in the future	Discuss contraception and the risks of unintended pregnancy
Before conception		Does the patient want to start or enlarge a family?
	Can I get pregnant?	Does the patient seek or need fertility treatment?
	Drugs during pregnancy and lactation	Adjust therapy to drugs compatible with pregnancy and lactation
During pregnancy	Will I get worse or better during pregnancy? Will I have more pregnancy complications than healthy women?	Inform on the interaction between pregnancy and the RD in question
	Will medications harm my baby?	Give balanced information on drugs during pregnancy
After delivery	Will the disease worsen after delivery?	Inform on the risk of relapse after delivery and necessity to restart therapy
	Can I use drugs during lactation?	Inform on drugs during breastfeeding
	Will I be able to care for children?	Refer patient to occupational therapist and physiotherapist

Severe lung disease, pulmonary arterial hypertension, severe cardiomyopathy, or renal insufficiency suggest discouraging pregnancy.

In the following, patient cases are presented together with key points of counselling. They deal with issues of fertility, assisted reproduction, drug switching, contradictory advice, conception at active disease, and comorbidities.

Case 1: Medications and fertility

A 34-year-old woman with a 4-year history of anti-citrullinated peptide antibodies (ACPA) positive rheumatoid arthritis (RA) complains of infertility. For 16 months she has unsuccessfully tried to conceive. Because of her wish for pregnancy, methotrexate (MTX) 20 mg weekly was discontinued 18 months ago and treatment with certolizumab pegol (CZP) was initiated. Despite CZP therapy, disease activity has not been optimally suppressed. During active periods the patient has taken additional prednisone with doses varying between 5–10 mg daily. At times of low disease activity, she has only taken ibuprofen 600 mg 2 times, sometimes 3 times a day. The patient is concerned that the previous MTX therapy has impaired her fertility. She also has read that ibuprofen and prednisone might disturb normal ovulation. She asks for referral to an infertility specialist.

Table 1.3 Interaction between pregnancy and different types of RD

Disease	Major clinical symptoms	Antiphospholipid antibodies (aPL); anti-Ro/-La present	Effect of pregnancy on disease activity	Pregnancy complications in the mother	Risk for adverse foetal/neonatal outcomes	Need for therapy during pregnancy
Rheumatoid arthritis	Arthritis	Rare	Improvement in 40–50% in RF[a] +, ACPA[b] + RA; 75% in ACPA, RF-RA	Increased at very active disease and comorbidities	Increased at very active disease and comorbidities	Continuation recommended for disease control. Dose reduction is possible
Ankylosing spondylitis	Spinal arthritis	No	Mostly unchanged compared to before pregnancy, flare around week 20	Increased at very active disease and comorbidities	Increased at very active disease and comorbidities	Continue effective therapy to prevent flare
Juvenile idiopathic arthritis	Subgroups* of arthritis and systemic disease	Rare	Poly- or pauci-arthritis often improve, Still's disease active	Increased at very active disease and comorbidities	Increased at very active disease and comorbidities	Need varies according to subtype
Psoriatic arthritis	Subgroups of arthritis	No	Variable according to subtype	Rare	Rare	Continuation recommended for disease control. Dose reduction is possible
Systemic lupus, erythematosus	Skin, arthritis, renal, haematological, CNS, serositis	aPL: 40% anti-Ro/-LA: 30%	Propensity to flare	Increased	Increased	Continue therapy for disease control. Treat flares effectively

Rare connective tissue diseases	Scleroderma; myositis + organ manifestations	Rare	Largely unaltered in established disease; aggravated at onset during pregnancy	Increased	Increased	Continue therapy for disease control. Treat flares effectively
Small vessel vasculitis	Pulmonary and renal	No	Insufficient data to make a statement	Increased	Increased	Continue therapy for disease control. Treat flares effectively
Antiphospholipid syndrome	Obstetric and thromboembolic events	aPL: 100%	Increased risk of thrombosis	Increased	Increased	Anticoagulation and anti-platelet therapy required

[a] rheumatoid factor; [b] anti-citrullinated protein antibodies; * subgroups of arthritis are mono-articular, pauci-articular or polyarticular and/or spinal arthritis.

Table 1.4 Risk assessment and stratification

Risk assessment		Risk stratification		
Risk factor	**Comment**	**Low risk**	**Medium risk***	**High risk**
Type of disease	Few organs involved or multi-organ disease	Predominant joint disease	Few non-vital organs involved	Multi-organ disease including kidney, heart, or lung
Stage of disease	New onset/early or established	Established and on stable medication	Established and on stable medication*	New onset/early disease
Disease activity	Recent or currently active	Low disease activity or remission	Low disease activity or remission*	Active disease at conception
Organ damage	Present in vital organs?	No organ damage	No or slight impairment of organ function	Irreversible organ damage present
Autoantibodies	Antiphospholipid antibodies (aPL); anti-Ro or -La rheumatoid factor and/or ACPA	No antibodies	Low titre aPL; rheumatoid factor and/or ACPA	Antiphospholipid antibodies and/or anti-Ro or -La
Comorbidities	Hypertension; diabetes; thyroid disease, APS; other	No comorbidities	None or one well-controlled comorbidity	APS and/or multiple comorbidities
Overweight	BMI > 25	Normal weight	Normal weight*	High BMI
Medications	Current treatment with embryo/foeto-toxic drugs	Therapy with pregnancy-compatible drugs	Therapy with pregnancy-compatible drugs*	Current treatment with embryo/foeto-toxic drugs
Recreational agents	Nicotine; alcohol, illicit drugs	No use	No use*	Use of nicotine or any recreational drug
Previous pregnancy complications	Gestational hypertension; gestational diabetes; pre-eclampsia, other adverse pregnancy outcomes	None	None*	History of any previous pregnancy complication

*Even in the absence of a particular risk factor but presence of any other risk factor, a medium risk may exist.

Case discussion

Population based studies show that there is reduced fertility and a reduced number of children in women with RD compared to their age matched peers. Reasons are multiple with failure to conceive, or impairment of implantation, or an increased rate of pregnancy losses (4). You can reassure the patient that low-dose MTX (5–30 mg/ weekly) does not impair female fertility. Studies assessing ovarian reserve by measuring anti-Müllerian hormone (AMH) have not found significant differences in AMH levels in patients with RA treated or not treated with MTX.

By contrast, chronic use of non-steroidal anti-inflammatory drugs (NSAIDs) can induce the luteinized unruptured follicle (LUF) syndrome by inhibiting the rupture of the follicle wall and release of the oocyte. However, treatment in the pre-ovulatory phase of the menstrual cycle with a full anti-inflammatory dose of an NSAID is required for this effect. Your patient has occasionally taken 1,200–1,800 mg of ibuprofen (full dose would be 2,400 mg/day) which in a study of women with RD and under continuous treatment with 1,200 mg ibuprofen did not induce LUF (5).

The influence of corticoids on fertility is debated due to concerns about confounding by indication, for example high disease activity, cannot be ruled out. Doses of 5–7.5 mg/day do probably not reduce fertility. High disease activity, however, reduces the chance to achieve a pregnancy within 12 months of unprotected intercourse. Your patient has not achieved remission or even stable low disease activity with the current treatment regimen, so a change of therapy should also be considered.

The referral to an infertility specialist is reasonable in this case. The patient needs to be aware that in up to 70% of RA patients no obvious cause for infertility can be found.

Case 2: Switching a patient from a teratogenic to a pregnancy-compatible drug

A 27-year-old woman developed a malar rash and arthralgias. Laboratory assessment showed positive antinuclear antibody (ANA), and double stranded deoxyribonucleic acid (dsDNA) antibodies. Three months later proteinuria, haematuria, and red cell casts in the urine were detected. Renal biopsy showed glomerulonephritis World Health Organization (WHO) class 4. The patient was treated with methylprednisolone pulses and IV cyclophosphamide (CYC) until in remission. She has continued with maintenance therapy with mycophenolate mofetil (MMF) 2 g/day. Lupus nephritis (LN) has been quiescent for the last 2 years. The patient is now 30 years old and wants a pregnancy. At her last consultation she reported a photosensitive rash 4 months ago, and arthritis in several finger joints 3 months ago. She has no active symptoms now and her blood pressure is normal. Laboratory results: normal renal function, dsDNA antibodies negative, and C3+C4 normal. Current therapy is hydroxychloroquine (HCQ) 400 mg/day, 5 mg prednisone/day, and MMF 2 g/day.

Case discussion

The patient had LN previously but has been in renal remission for the last 2 years. She had minor lupus symptoms recently but is without symptoms now and her laboratory tests are normal. However, pregnancy must be postponed because of therapy with MMF. The patient should be advised to taper and discontinue MMF. Subsequently she will be transferred to azathioprine (AZA), which she can take throughout pregnancy (6) (see Chapter 3.1). During an observation time of 6 months renal function and activity will be monitored to ensure that remission of LN is maintained after the transitioning from MMF to AZA. During the observation time birth control should be practised.

Several highly effective drugs are teratogenic and not compatible with pregnancy including MTX, CYC, and mycophenolate derivatives (see Chapter 3.2). This underlines the necessity to address family planning whenever a patient is started on any of these drugs in order to avoid pregnancies occurring under therapy with a teratogenic drug. In addition, advice on effective contraception (effective regarding prevention of conception) must be routinely given to patients on treatment with teratogenic drugs. Natural and barrier methods are highly unreliable and only hormonal contraceptives, intrauterine devices (IUD), and sterilization have acceptable efficacy with low failure rates (7). Hormonal oestrogen-containing contraceptives should be avoided in women with a high-risk profile of phospholipid antibodies (high titre or triple positivity) or antiphospholipid syndrome (APS). If the treating rheumatologist lacks experience to counsel on contraception, referral to a gynaecologist is indicated. The consistency of contraceptive use should be checked repeatedly.

Case 3: Contradictory advice on medication

A 30-year-old woman has suffered from systemic lupus erythematosus (SLE) for seven years with main symptoms from the skin, arthritis, and cytopenia. Her immunological profile includes high titre ANA, positivity for anti-Sjögren's-syndrome-related antigen A (SSA), and anti-Sjögren's-syndrome-related antigen B (SSB), medium titre IgG cardiolipin antibodies, and normal complement levels. The childless patient has consulted her rheumatologist because of a wish to start a family. It was agreed that she should continue during pregnancy her medication consisting of HCQ 200 mg × 2/day, AZA 2 mg/kg/day, and prednisone 5 mg/day which she has tolerated well, and which have kept her disease under control.

At the next visit the patient tells the rheumatologist that she is pregnant in gestational week 13. She has seen her obstetrician at week 7 of pregnancy and he has told her to stop both HCQ and AZA immediately, but that she might continue low-dose prednisone. When seeing her general practitioner for a urinary tract infection, he has told her to continue HCQ, but to stop AZA throughout pregnancy. The patient is confused by the contradictory advice and fears that she perhaps has harmed her baby by taking HCQ and AZA during the first 6 weeks of her pregnancy.

Case discussion

The case reveals a frequent problem: pregnant women have multiple HCP and may get different advice regarding their treatment during pregnancy. HCP not familiar with the course and prognosis of SLE may be reticent to continue necessary medications.

Communication with all HCP involved (obstetricians, other medical specialists, midwives, and specialist nurses) in an individual patient's care early on is necessary in order to avoid conflicting advice which is confusing and distressing for the patient and may lead to discontinuation of all medications. Communication with other HCP should emphasize that inadequate treatment of maternal disease compromises foetal wellbeing. Abrupt stop of effective drugs may result in a relapse and worsening of the maternal disease.

Lack of optimal communication and of shared care is a frequent problem between specialists. It is prudent to give a brief management plan including information for the indication of treatment to the patient so she can show it to other HCP involved in her care.

Time should also be spent with the patient to fully discuss the relative safety of each individual medication, and the comparative risks of undertreated autoimmune, or inflammatory disease. She should be assured that her concerns are valid and that differing recommendations add anxiety to her decision making. She should be armed with as much information as possible and encouraged to reach out when concern or anxiety arises. Often, spending time discussing pregnancy concerns with the patient and her partner or other close family members can help understanding of the specific issues related to her given situation.

Case 4: Conception at active early disease

A 24-year-old woman has recently immigrated from another country to Europe. She has basic education but does not speak a European language. Her husband works as an engineer and speaks English reasonably well. The couple has three small daughters of 1, 2.5, and 4 years. Two months after the birth of the last child she developed arthritis in several MCP and PIP joints, the right wrist, and in several metatarso-phalangeal (MTP) joints of the feet. The general practitioner found elevated erythrocyte sedimentation rate (ESR) and C-reactive protein (CRP), low haemoglobin, positivity for rheumatoid factor, and for ACPA, and referred her to a rheumatologist. At the first rheumatology visit, the patient met with a translator. Ultrasound examination showed several early erosions in finger joints and two MTP joints. Disease activity score (DAS) was 5.8. The diagnosis of seropositive RA was made and explained to the patient. Therapy with 20 mg MTX weekly and 10 mg of prednisone was suggested as a start of a treat-to-target (T2T) management plan. The patient refused and explained that she wanted to have a new pregnancy soon, and that she hopes the next child will be a son. She does not agree to medications but prefers herbal medicine.

Case discussion

The patient has new onset seropositive RA. Risk assessment reveals several predictors for progressive disease: ACPA positivity, early erosions, and high DAS. Pregnancy at this stage would be ill-timed. Risk stratification in this patient shows high risk for active maternal disease and risk for prematurity and intrauterine growth restriction (IUGR) in the child because of systemic maternal inflammation. Prompt start of effective therapy to control inflammation and prevent further joint damage is mandatory in her case. The best advice would be to postpone pregnancy until low disease activity or remission is achieved.

Several challenges for optimal communication must be overcome in this case. Therefore, a new appointment should be made with the patient and her husband together. Diagnosis and future development of RA should be explained to the couple. They need to understand the chronic and progressive nature of RA and the risk of functional disability in case no therapy is initiated. Herbal medicine will not be able to control active RA. The couple's wish of a fourth pregnancy may be threatened by high maternal disease activity. It is actually in their own interest and for the benefit of a future child to control disease activity effectively before attempting a pregnancy. In case counselling fails to convince the couple to postpone their pregnancy wish every attempt must be made to convince them of the necessity to start a pregnancy-compatible and fast-acting drug right away. The best option for this patient would be initiation of a tumor necrosis factor (TNF) inhibitor with low placental passage. In general, biologics with a low placental passage should be prescribed to any patient of fertile age with a future pregnancy in view.

It is evident that counselling a case like this is time consuming. In a time with limited budgets, constrained resources, and overburdened HCP finding time for comprehensive counselling is difficult. It may help to share the task with other members of the rheumatology team like rheumatology specialist nurses.

Case 5: Ro/La positive mother

A 33-year-old mother has been diagnosed with undifferentiated connective tissue disease (UCTD) 5 years ago. She has mild symptoms including keratoconjunctivitis sicca and xerostomia. Her autoantibody profile shows elevated titres of anti-Ro52 antibodies and anti-La antibodies. The patient has a pregnancy wish and has searched the internet for information on anti-Ro/-La antibodies. She became alarmed when reading about CHB. She contacts her rheumatologist to discuss the prospect and the risk of a future pregnancy. She also wishes to know whether there is any prophylactic treatment for prevention of CHB.

Case discussion

CHB is a foetal cardiac injury, detected before, at birth, or within the neonatal period caused by transplacental passage of maternal antibodies against SS-A/Ro and SS-B/La ribonucleoproteins (see Chapter 2.4). The incidence of CHB in children of a mother with the pathological autoantibodies ranges between 1.6–2%, in other words it is a rare event. However, a complete 3rd degree atrioventricular (AV) block is serious and requires a pacemaker after birth. Therefore, screening of the foetal heart rate starting at week 16 and stopping at week 28 is recommended in anti-Ro/SSA positive women by most experts (8, 9). These are the basic facts the patient needs to know.

Unfortunately, no consensus exists on the frequency and the mode of screening. In patients with SLE, Sjøgren, or UCTD the proportion of anti-Ro/SSA positive women is up to 40%. Monitoring all these women with weekly foetal echocardiograms (echo) during pregnancy requires expert and financial resources that are not available in every country or every hospital. For women without a prior infant with CHB, weekly auscultatory heart rate monitoring done with a hand-held Doppler during week 16–28 is an adequate option. If the heart rate is normal, then a CHB is excluded. In case of dysrhythmia (bradycardia, arrhythmia) the mother should be referred for an echo.

The general risk after birth of a CHB child to have a recurrence is 17.4%. Cardiac neonatal lupus (NLE) can overlap with skin NLE. After birth of a child with skin rash the risk increases 12–16% to have a child with CHB in the next pregnancy. Women with a prior infant with neonatal lupus should have weekly foetal echos during weeks 16–28. After birth the neonate should have an ECG, which should be repeated several times during the first year of life.

Prevention of CHB has been tried in different ways. Prophylactic therapy in mothers positive for anti-SSA/B but without a prior child with CHB or NLE is not indicated. When varying degrees of atrioventricular (AV) block are detected during screening, most experts would start dexa- or beta-methasone either for preventing progress of AV block degree I or II to a complete block or at signs of cardiomyopathy. The duration of therapy with fluorinated corticoids and their efficacy is debated. There is no robust evidence that they actually can reverse AV block. One needs to remember that they are not without toxicity for the mother and foetus. Intravenous immuno-globulin has not proven to effectively prevent recurrence of CHB.

Several publications found a reduction of CHB recurrence as well as lower occur-rence of NLE in women using HCQ during pregnancy. An international study on prevention of a recurrence of CHB (PATCH) by treatment with HCQ is ongoing but results have not been published yet. HCQ is a drug that has few side effects and is tol-erated well by most patients, which supports its use during pregnancy in women with a previous NLE or CHB child. However, during counselling one must make it clear that success of HCQ is not guaranteed.

Informing anti-Ro/SSA positive women about the significance of the antibodies re-quires psychological skill. The threat of possible heart disease in a baby feels alarming for the mother and may stress her throughout pregnancy. Therefore, it must be pointed out that CHB is a rather unlikely event, but that screening is desirable in all pregnant women positive for the antibodies. Most experts would recommend HCQ during pregnancy in all anti-Ro/SSA positive women.

Case 6: Patient with obesity and comorbidities

A 39-year-old childless woman with psoriatic arthritis (PsA) affecting both knees, the right ankle, and periodically the elbow joints plans a pregnancy. Her skin disease is located on the scalp, around the abdomen, and the gluteal region. She is obese with a BMI of 34 and smokes 5–10 cigarettes daily. She has been treated with enalapril 20 mg × 2/day and amlodipine 10 mg/day the last 4 years for hypertension. The patient has undergone several attempts of assisted reproduction treatment (ART) in the last 3 years without success. She contacts her rheumatologist for advice on how to improve her prospect of becoming a mother.

Case discussion

The present patient has several factors that decrease fertility: age, obesity, chronic disease, and smoking. Female fertility decreases with age with a marked decrease of ovarian follicles after age 30. Chronic inflammation like PsA can diminish ovarian reserve further. Obesity impairs the hormonal balance and results in ovulatory dysfunction which lowers the success rate of ART procedures. In addition, obese women are at risk for medical complications during pregnancy such as miscarriage, gestational hypertension, pre-eclampsia, and gestational diabetes. Obese pregnant women also have an increased rate of Caesarean section. There is even an increased risk of congenital malformations and foetal macrosomia independent of any medication exposure. The negative effects of smoking on fertility and pregnancy and child outcome are well documented.

Lifestyle factors must be reviewed pre-conceptionally and be adjusted to the benefit of pregnancy. A change of lifestyle is urgently needed in this patient, therefore she should be referred to a registered dietitian for counselling about weight loss, nutrition, and food choices. The patient should be encouraged to lose weight before conception and enter pregnancy with a BMI <30 kg/m^2, ideally <25 kg/m^2. Regular physical activity may help to achieve this goal. Moderate to vigorous physical activity for 2–3 hours each week spread over at least 3 days with no more than 2 consecutive inactive days would be of benefit. In addition to consuming a healthy diet, the patient should be advised to stop smoking immediately.

Management: Drug treatment needs to be adjusted. The patient takes an ACE inhibitor for hypertension. ACE inhibitors are foetotoxic when administered in the 2nd and 3rd trimester, therefore she needs to switch from enalapril to another antihypertensive (see Chapter 3.1) but not before a pregnancy test is positive. After the switch, weekly control of blood pressure should be done.

Case 7: Assisted reproduction in a woman with phospholipid antibodies

A 37-year-old woman without children has had two early pregnancy miscarriages. Laboratory tests have shown positivity for anticardiolipin antibodies, β2-glycoprotein I antibodies, and lupus anticoagulant at repeated testing. She has no clinical or laboratory signs of SLE and had no thrombotic event previously. After the last miscarriage the patient has not become pregnant again despite trying to conceive. She wants to undergo assisted reproduction with in vitro fertilization (IVF).

Case discussion

The patient had two miscarriages and is triple positive for aPL. Despite this finding she does not fill the current classification criteria for APS which require three or more consecutive 1st trimester miscarriages in addition to persistent aPL. Until now she had no clinical symptoms, particularly no thrombosis. ART procedures include ovarian stimulation, oocyte retrieval, IVF, and transfer of the fertilized embryo into the uterus. The question is whether the patient should receive prophylactic anticoagulation treatment.

Prophylactic antithrombotic therapy during IVF for women with aPL without APS but with risk factors is recommended (11). The presence of aPL alone does not appear to adversely affect pregnancy rates or outcome in patients who are undergoing IVF. However, the patient has several risk factors (age and triple aPL positivity) that might suggest following the guidelines given for patients with SLE and APS despite the absence of these diagnoses (10). This includes mild ovarian stimulation, a protocol avoiding ovarian hyperstimulation, single frozen embryo transfer in a natural cycle, and luteal phase support. Low-dose aspirin and prophylactic doses of low-molecular-weight heparin should be administered during ovarian stimulation, pregnancy, and 6 weeks postpartum according the European League Against Rheumatism (EULAR) recommendations for ART and pregnancy in women with SLE and/or APS (8).

Recent studies confirm the relative safety of ART in patients with SLE and/or APS. IVF procedures have not shown an increased risk for thrombosis when SLE and APS are clinically quiescent and controlled by medications. Whether the presence of aPL or APS influences the number of required IVF cycles has been debated. There is, however, no indication of reduced fertility success rates.

General recommendations for pre-conception counselling

The best chance to achieve shared patient–clinician decision making through counselling is to build a personal relationship supported by mutual trust. The HCP needs to listen carefully to all concerns around pregnancy and child rearing the patient may have, which gives the clinician a better understanding of the patient's reservations, and allows an opportunity to clarify misconceptions. Ideally, the partner or a family member of the patient should be present at counselling. They can help the woman to make the right decisions regarding family planning and adjustment of therapy.

The clinician should consider how to communicate the individual patient's disease-related or medication-related risks in a way that is realistic and reassuring. Ideally counselling should be offered by an experienced HCP who gives a balanced account of the risks and prognosis of a future pregnancy, and discusses treatment options, as well as management and monitoring during and after pregnancy.

Drug therapy

Medications during pregnancy and lactation are a major concern of patients planning a pregnancy. Many women would rather suffer a flare than expose their baby to any harm by therapy. Counselling must inform the patient that untreated maternal disease increases the risk for adverse pregnancy outcome. It is important to explain to the patient that continuing pregnancy-compatible drugs helps to maintain remission or low disease activity and prevent a flare or organ damage. Beneficial effects in the child are prevention of miscarriage, intrauterine growth restriction, and premature delivery, as well as reducing problems with parenting after delivery. Pre-term delivery, even if relatively late in gestation, can have long-term adverse health consequences for the child throughout childhood and into adulthood, even in the absence of any congenital malformations. Information on drug treatment during pregnancy and lactation needs to consider the patient's values, preferences, and circumstances. Patients who are well informed and involved in treatment decisions are more likely to adhere to a management plan and to therapy.

Control of disease activity is the most important indication for medications. If changes of therapy are necessary, for example because of teratogenicity, these changes should be made well in advance of a planned pregnancy to be sure the new medication regimen effectively controls the underlying disease. If one does not know whether a patient is planning a pregnancy, one should treat her as if she were.

Interdisciplinary communication and coordinated care

HCP from different specialties must fulfil various tasks including recognizing high-risk pregnancy, performing pre-conception assessment and counselling, providing monitoring, and management throughout pregnancy and ensuring that a post-partum flare is avoided. The need for collaboration and dialogue is often impeded because of lack of consensus. The scarcity of dialogue between rheumatologists, general practitioners, obstetricians, and pharmacists may negatively impact the adequacy of the care of a pregnant patient. Most often inconsistencies of advice to the patient or different approaches to the care of pregnant women confuse the patient. The rheumatologist involved in pre-conception and pregnancy care should therefore actively seek communication and collaboration with the other HCP caring for patients during pregnancy.

Key messages

- It's the task of the HCP to actively address family planning.
- Good counselling focuses on the individual patient and her fertility goals.
- Counselling is based on risk assessment and risk stratification in the individual patient.
- Contraception counselling is mandatory when prescribing potentially teratogenic drugs, and in patients with active disease, or severe organ damage.
- Give information that enables the patient to make informed decisions on management during pregnancy and lactation.
- Communication and collaboration with other HCP who already are or will be involved in pregnancy management support coordinated care.

Further reading

1. Østensen M. Preconception counseling. *Rheum Dis Clin North Am*. 2017;43(2):189–99.
2. Andreoli L, Lazzaroni MG, Carini C, Dall'Ara F, Nalli C, Reggia R, Rodrigues M, et al. 'Disease knowledge index' and perspectives on reproductive issues: A nationwide study on 398 women with autoimmune rheumatic diseases. *Joint Bone Spine*. 2018;pii:S1297–319X(18)30257–4.

3. Ackerman IN, Ngian GS, Van Doornum S, Briggs AM. A systematic review of interventions to improve knowledge and self-management skills concerning contraception, pregnancy and breastfeeding in people with rheumatoid arthritis. *Clin Rheumatol.* 2016;35(1):33–41.

4. Østensen M. Sexual and reproductive health in rheumatic disease. *Nat Rev Rheumatol.* 2017;13(8):485–93.

5. Micu MC, Micu R, Ostensen M. Luteinized unruptured follicle syndrome increased by inactive disease and selective cyclooxygenase 2 inhibitors in women with inflammatory arthropathies. *Arthritis Care Res* (Hoboken). 2011;63(9):1334–38.

6. Fischer-Betz R, Specker C, Brinks R, Aringer M, Schneider M. Low risk of renal flares and negative outcomes in women with lupus nephritis conceiving after switching from mycophenolate mofetil to azathioprine. *Rheumatology* (Oxford). 2013;52(6):1070–76.

7. Sammaritano LR. Contraception in patients with rheumatic disease. *Rheum Dis Clin North Am.* 2017;43(2):173–18.

8. Andreoli L, Bertsias GK, Agmon-Levin N, S Brown S, Cervera R, Costedoat-Chalumeau N, et al. EULAR recommendations for women's health and the management of family planning, assisted reproduction, pregnancy and menopause in patients with systemic lupus erythematosus and/or antiphospholipid syndrome. *Ann Rheum Dis.* 2017;76:476–85.

9. Clowse MEB, Eudy AM, Kiernan E, Williams MR, Bermas B, Chakravarty E, Sammaritano LR, Chambers CD, Buyon J. The prevention, screening and treatment of congenital heart block from neonatal lupus: A survey of provider practices. *Rheumatology* (Oxford). 2018;57(suppl_5):v9–v17.

10. Bellver J, Pellicer A. Ovarian stimulation for ovulation induction and in vitro fertilization in patients with systemic lupus erythematosus and antiphospholipid syndrome. *Fertil Steril.* 2009;92:1803–10.

11. Tektonidou MG, Andreoli L, Limper M, Amoura Z, Cervera R, Costedoat-Chalumeau N, et al. EULAR recommendations for the management of antiphospholipid syndrome in adults. *Ann Rheum Dis.* 2019 May 15. pii: annrheumdis-2019-215213. doi: 10.1136/annrheumdis-2019-215213. [Epub ahead of print].

SECTION II
PATIENTS WITH PRE-PREGNANCY COMPLICATIONS

2.1

Thrombotic complications in pregnant patients with rheumatic disease

Andrew James Doyle and Beverley Jane Hunt

Case 1: Management of a patient with RA and previous thrombosis during pregnancy

A 27-year-old woman was diagnosed with a deep vein thrombosis (DVT) and pulmonary embolism (PE) following a 2-week history of right lower limb pain and a 2-day history of pleuritic chest pain and dyspnea. In her past medical history, she had been diagnosed with rheumatoid arthritis (RA) aged 24 years. She had a DAS28 score of 2.2 indicating well-controlled disease at the time of venous thromboembolism (VTE) diagnosis, which was treated with intermittent non-steroidal anti-inflammatories (NSAIDs). She had no previous pregnancies and was not using oestrogen-containing contraception. No other provoking factors for VTE were identified. Her family history was notable only for a mother who had DVT following the birth of her third child.

Inherited thrombophilia testing and antiphospholipid antibodies (aPL) testing was performed and were normal. She was treated as having an unprovoked VTE and commenced on rivaroxaban 15 mg twice daily for 3 weeks then long-term rivaroxaban 20 mg once daily. She suffered from menorrhagia, which was treated with tranexamic acid during her menses and the dose of rivaroxaban was reduced to 10 mg after 6 months.

She became pregnant at the age of 31 years and was changed from rivaroxaban (see Chapter 3.1) to low-molecular-weight heparin (LMWH) 5,000 units once daily (prophylactic dose) after a positive pregnancy test. She was advised to stop taking NSAIDs. The pregnancy progressed well with normal growth scans, blood pressure, and urinalysis. At 32 weeks' gestation, she developed acute central chest pain. Bilateral leg compression ultrasonography was performed, which was unremarkable, and a subsequent computed tomography pulmonary angiography (CTPA) did not show a PE; anti-Xa was at a peak level and within expected ranges. She was treated as having acute costochondritis and responded to paracetamol and dihydrocodeine (see Chapter 3.1). She continued the same dose of LMWH until delivery. She delivered at 39 weeks with a spontaneous vaginal delivery requiring inhaled nitrous oxide only for analgesia. There was no significant bleeding postpartum and she delivered a healthy 3-kg baby. She breastfed, so was restarted on LMWH 12-hours post-delivery and switched to warfarin with a target international normalized ratio (INR) of 2–3 until breastfeeding ceased. She restarted rivaroxaban when no longer breastfeeding.

Case discussion

This case highlights the management of a woman with a previous history of VTE who becomes pregnant with a background of RA. There was the concern of a recurrent VTE in her 3rd trimester, but subsequent imaging was negative.

Thrombosis in pregnancy

VTE occurs in 0.6–1.2 of every 10,000 pregnancies and is the most common direct cause of maternal death in the United Kingdom in approximately 1 in 100,000 pregnancies (1). Therefore, the recognition of mothers at high risk of VTE is imperative.

Pregnancy is a prothrombotic state that begins at conception lasting to 6–12 weeks postpartum. There is 4–6-fold increased risk of VTE in pregnancy compared with age-matched controls. There are physiological increases in the levels of fibrinogen, prothrombin, factors VII and VIII, and von Willebrand factor (vWF); reduced levels of the natural anticoagulant, protein S; and altered activity of the fibrinolytic system. These changes are thought to allow adequate haemostasis at the time of delivery. These changes as well as changes in blood flow in the legs and altered endothelial function of pregnancy contribute to the risk of VTE. The use of preconceptual oestrogen as part of in vitro fertilization, maternal obesity, increasing age, multiparity, and smoking can further increase thrombotic risks. Transient prothrombotic risk factors in pregnancy include hyperemesis gravidarum, dehydration, sepsis, immobility, and surgical procedures during pregnancy including Caesarean section. Inherited thrombophilias such as antithrombin deficiency have higher rates of thrombosis during this period.

The clinical nature of DVT in pregnancy is different from that outside of pregnancy. They are typically left-sided (72%), occur in the proximal leg veins, and 42% of women develop post-thrombotic syndrome. May–Thurner syndrome is the compression to venous outflow of the left common iliac vein when it is transversed by the right iliac artery at the level of the fifth lumbar vertebra. This can be further compressed by the gravid uterus at this level and is a contributing factor to pregnancy-related VTE.

Thrombosis in inflammatory and rheumatic diseases

Inflammatory conditions, such as systemic lupus erythematosus (SLE), dermatomyositis, RA, and inflammatory bowel disease (IBD), have higher rates of thrombosis particularly at the time of diagnosis and with active disease. This is partly due to increased levels of procoagulant acute phase proteins particularly prothrombin, VWF, FVIII, and fibrinogen. Hospitalization or immobilization of patients with these conditions can further contribute to this risk.

The presence of aPL is a risk factor for thromboembolism and associated with other autoimmune conditions. They are estimated to be present in 30–40% of patients with SLE and around 28% with RA, compared to 1–5% of the general population. The presence of repeatedly positive aPL in addition to thromboembolic or specific obstetric manifestations is known as antiphospholipid syndrome (APS).

Rates of VTE during pregnancy in women with autoimmune diseases including SLE, RA, IBD, and dermatomyositis are higher than those without. Given the prothrombotic risk of both pregnancy and inflammatory disease, these conditions are recognized as a risk factor for VTE in pregnancy and are included as part of the Royal College of Obstetricians risk stratification tool (2).

Diagnosis of VTE during pregnancy

Current practice for diagnosis of VTE outside of pregnancy is dependent on using clinical pre-test probability scoring tools, such as the Wells score, in combination with D-dimer, a fibrin-degradation product, in those with clinical features of VTE. Those with a low-risk score require no further imaging whereas those with high-risk scores require compression ultrasonography (US) for the diagnosis of DVT and if patients have symptoms of pulmonary embolism (PE) then CTPA or ventilation/perfusion (V/Q) scanning are required.

In pregnancy, several issues arise with this model of diagnosis for there had been inadequate studies to assess the utility of pre-test probability scores and D-dimer. This has resulted in pregnant women being sent for imaging without risk assessment and D-dimer testing. As some of the symptoms and signs of DVT and PE are difficult to distinguish from the physiological changes of pregnancy, many women are sent for scanning, and studies show that the positive diagnostic rate of CTPA in pregnancy is only 2–3%. Two recent studies have looked at the utility of pre-test probability testing in the diagnosis of PE in pregnancy. Righini et al. (7) used the modified Geneva risk score and D-dimer and van De Pol et al. (6) used a modified form of the YEARS score (simplified diagnostic management of suspected pulmonary embolism prospective cohort study (the YEARS study)) with D-dimer. They both concluded that their assessment would exclude PE adequately. But both studies have been criticized for having inadequate safety margins and would miss some cases of PE, which could be catastrophic. Furthermore, the findings are in conflict with the diagnosis of PE in pregnancy study (DiPEP, 3), a prospective cohort study, where clinical prediction scores and D-dimer were shown to have no utility. Further studies are necessary to look at this area. Therefore, at present pregnant women with clinical features of VTE should undergo diagnostic imaging without clinical scoring or D-dimer testing.

DVT can be assessed easily and rapidly using Doppler compression ultrasound (CUS) looking for a thrombus although it must be remembered that this test is dependent on an experienced operator and thromboses can be missed. National Institute for Health and Care Excellence (NICE) recommend CUS above the popliteal fossa due to their higher risk of embolization than those below this level (4). The procedure is non-invasive, affordable, and does not risk damage to the mother or foetus. Repeat imaging may however be required if clinical suspicion remains high with a negative initial test.

Imaging for PE during pregnancy can prove more challenging. All should have CUS first to avoid unnecessary radiation and, if negative, CTPA or V/Q imaging should be performed. CTPA has been associated with an increased risk of maternal breast cancer whereas V/Q imaging can cause slight increased risk of childhood cancer although the absolute risk of both complications is very small. V/Q scan is preferred in women with a family history of breast cancer and previous chest computed tomography (CT) imaging. Such rare risks should be discussed with mothers before imaging; however, imaging should not be avoided or delayed as there is a significantly higher risk of maternal mortality from an undiagnosed and untreated PE.

Management of anticoagulation in pregnancy

For those who present with a VTE during pregnancy, anticoagulation should be started with the clinical suspicion of a VTE and continued or stopped depending on confirmatory imaging. LMWH is the preferred anticoagulant during pregnancy; and those diagnosed with a pregnancy-related VTE should have anticoagulation continued for at least 6 weeks postpartum or a minimum of 3 months of treatment in total. This should be based upon the woman's early pregnancy weight and can be given as once or twice daily injections. Women should also be assessed for renal impairment and, if present, LMWH doses should be adjusted accordingly. Subcutaneous unfractionated heparin (UFH) can be used when LMWH is not available although it requires an increased frequency of injections. Vitamin K antagonists (VKA) such as warfarin should not be used during pregnancy due to the 2% risk of foetal warfarin syndrome in the 1st trimester, which can cause skeletal malformation, cognitive impairment, and deafness, and increased foetal bleeding risk in the 2nd and 3rd trimester because it crosses the placenta. Direct oral anticoagulants (DOAC) including rivaroxaban, apixaban, edoxaban, and dabigatran (see Chapter 3.1) have little current safety data in humans and have shown adverse outcome in animal models in pregnancy so are currently not advised. Intravenous UFH is typically reserved for women who have a high bleeding risk but need to continue anticoagulation during labour.

For those who are taking anticoagulation pre-pregnancy such as this patient, some guidelines recommend switching a DOAC to LMWH pre-conceptually, but we recommend oral anticoagulation should be stopped when a positive pregnancy test is obtained and changed to LMWH. Prenatally, these women should be counselled about the increased risk of thrombosis in pregnancy and the need for LMWH as well as discussion of lifestyle modifications such as smoking cessation, weight loss, and stopping alcohol consumption. The dosing of LMWH for those on long-term anticoagulation during pregnancy is dependent of the history and site of previous thrombosis and is described in Table 2.1.1. Dose increases in LMWH may be required after 16 weeks due to the increased plasma volume of pregnancy, which increases by 40%, and an increased physiological clearance of heparin in the later stages of pregnancy.

Routine monitoring of anticoagulation is not required during pregnancy in most patients due to the predictable pharmacokinetics of LMWH. Women at the extremes of weight (<50 kg or >90 kg), or those with complicating factors such as recurrence of VTE whilst on LMWH, or renal impairment with a creatinine clearance <15 ml/min, require monitoring. Those with antithrombin deficiency should be managed by a haematologist for their regular monitoring, and usually require very large doses of LMWH because LMWH acts by potentiating antithrombin. In the presence of low levels of antithrombin, higher doses of LMWH are required. Anti-Xa levels are taken

Table 2.1.1 Management of anticoagulation in pregnancy

Scenario	Treatment
Previous pregnancy-related VTE	Prophylactic dose LMWH from conception
Previous non-pregnancy-related VTE	Change from DOAC or VKA to LMWH from conception Prophylactic LMWH if single VTE Immediate/high-dose LMWH if recurrent VTE or arterial thrombosis
Active pregnancy-related VTE	Once or twice daily treatment-dose LMWH for 3 months or 6 weeks postpartum

DOAC—direct oral anticoagulant; LMWH—low-molecular-weight heparin; VKA—vitamin K antagonist; VTE—venous thromboembolism.

2–4 hours following administration for a peak level and immediately prior to subsequent dosing for a trough level.

It is imperative that a delivery plan is devised in conjunction with all responsible clinical teams as early as possible before or during pregnancy in order to reduce the risk of postpartum haemorrhage or thrombotic complications, and optimize analgesia management. If a spontaneous vaginal delivery is planned, women should be advised to stop LMWH when amniotic membranes rupture and/or uterine contractions are established. For elective Caesarean sections and induced deliveries, neuraxial analgesia such as epidural catheters should not be performed until at least 12 hours from the last administration of prophylactic dose LMWH and at least 24 hours for therapeutic doses due to the risk of vertebral canal haematoma. LMWH should not be given for at least 4 hours after an epidural catheter has been inserted or removed. The catheters should not be removed until at least 12 hours after the last administration of LMWH.

Inferior vena cava (IVC) filters are not routinely advised in pregnancy-related VTE except in a small number of women who have had VTE within a short time period prior to delivery (typically 2 weeks or less) with evidence of proximal DVT that may embolize. Previous VTE is not an indication for Caesarean section unless there are other obstetric or medical reasons. Following delivery, anticoagulation can be restarted once haemostasis is achieved. Both VKA and LMWH can be used safely when breastfeeding (those on VKAs are recommended to ensure that their neonates have adequate vitamin K) although DOAC cannot be used as there is inadequate safety data.

Case 2: A patient with cerebral antiphospholipid syndrome

A 25-year-old woman presented with left-sided weakness and slurred speech and was found to have a right parietal infarct on CT. aPL serology testing showed an IgG anticardiolipin antibody level of 78 U/L and lupus anticoagulant positive by DRVVT although anti-B2GP antibodies were negative. Other investigations for the stroke, including 24-hour cardiac monitoring and bubble echocardiogram, were normal. She was subsequently diagnosed with thrombotic aPL syndrome after subsequent positive aPL tests were performed 12 weeks later. She was started on warfarin with target INR 3–4 and did not suffer from significant menorrhagia.

She became pregnant aged 28 years old. She was immediately changed to dalteparin 5,000 units twice daily, and aspirin 75 mg once daily. She developed itching and hives around the dalteparin injection sites within 2 weeks of starting, so was changed to enoxaparin that she tolerated. Her platelet counts remained within normal limits. Uterine artery Doppler velocimetry performed at 20 weeks showed normal resistive indices and no notching. Urinalysis and blood pressure were normal throughout her pregnancy.

The obstetricians opted for a vaginal delivery, which was performed using spinal anaesthesia. The patient's LMWH was stopped 24 hours pre-procedure and a healthy girl weighing 3.2 kg was delivered. Post-operatively there was an estimated blood loss of 1 liter postpartum within the first 2 hours. Intravenous tranexamic acid was given, and bleeding settled. Twelve hours post-procedure, a prophylactic dose of enoxaparin was introduced and was continued after a further 24 hours and warfarin was restarted.

Case discussion

This case highlights a woman who presented with an ischaemic stroke who was diagnosed with APS. On becoming pregnant, she was anticoagulated with dalteparin but developed dalteparin allergy. This did not occur with enoxaparin. She had regular monitoring to assess for adverse obstetric outcomes. Post-delivery, she had a small postpartum haemorrhage and was managed accordingly.

Clinical features and presentation of antiphospholipid syndrome

APS is an autoimmune condition characterized by the presence of aPL of which the most clinically relevant are the lupus anticoagulant, anticardiolipin antibodies, and anti-β_2- glycoprotein-I antibodies. It can either occur alone or be associated with the presence of other autoimmune disorders. The mechanism by which aPL cause thrombosis is uncertain. Studies suggest activation of coagulation, complement activation via the classical pathway, impaired fibrinolysis, and activated protein C resistance (5). It has an estimated incidence of 5 per 100,000 people per year and a prevalence of 40–50 per 100,000. Autoimmunity is typically found in the family history of around 5% of patients with APS. The condition presents either as a thrombosis or adverse obstetric outcomes. The latter will be discussed further in Chapter 8. The classification criteria are dependent on the presence of both clinical features and laboratory findings shown in Table 2.1.2.

In contrast to inherited thrombophilias which predispose to VTE, APS can cause thrombi in veins, arteries, or microvasculature, also known as thrombotic microangiopathy (TMA). The most common arterial events are neurological presenting with ischaemic stroke or transient ischaemic attacks (TIA) whereas venous events are DVT and PE. Other sites of infarcts or presentations include cardiac

COUNSELLING, MONITORING, AND ASSESSMENT 27

Table 2.1.2 The Sydney criteria for antiphospholipid syndrome (APS)

Vascular thrombosis:	≥1 clinical episode of arterial, venous, or small vessel thrombosis. Thrombosis must be objectively confirmed. For histopathological confirmation, thrombosis must be present without inflammation of the vessel wall.
Pregnancy morbidity:	1. ≥1 unexplained death of a morphologically normal foetus ≥10 weeks of gestation (late miscarriage). 2. ≥1 premature delivery of a morphologically normal foetus <34 weeks gestation because of adverse obstetric outcomes: • severe pre-eclampsia or eclampsia defined according to standard definition; • recognized features of placental insufficiency. 3. ≥3 unexplained consecutive miscarriages <10 weeks gestation (early miscarriage), with maternal and paternal factors (anatomic, hormonal, or chromosomal abnormalities) excluded.
Laboratory criteria:	The presence of aPL, on two or more occasions at least 12 weeks apart and no more than five years prior to clinical manifestations, as demonstrated by ≥1 of the following: a. presence of lupus anticoagulant in plasma; b. medium to high-titre anticardiolipin antibodies (>40GPL or MPL, or >99th percentile) of IgG or IgM isoforms; c. anti-β2 glycoprotein-I antibody (anti-β_2GP I) of IgG or IgM present in plasma.

aPL—antiphospholipid antibodies; APS—antiphospholipid syndrome.

arteries, retinal veins/arteries, renal vessels, or TMA, vascular dementia, bony infarcts, and splanchnic veins. Non-thrombotic associations of APS are livedo reticularis (20% of patients), arthropathy, thrombocytopenia (20% of patients which is usually non-severe), autoimmune haemolytic anaemia, and Libman-Sacks endocarditis, a fibrin-rich deposition on heart valves although they are normally asymptomatic.

aPL testing should be performed a minimum of 12 weeks apart to confirm the persistence of the antibodies, which can be transiently positive at times of infection or inflammation. Patients with positive results for all three tests are said to have 'triple-positive' APS and have the highest rates of thrombosis and pregnancy-related complications. Patients with triple-positive antibodies have a risk of developing thrombosis of 12.2%, 26.1%, and 44.2% after 1, 5, and 10 years respectively.

Counselling, monitoring, and assessment of antiphospholipid syndrome during pregnancy

Women diagnosed with either APS presenting with thromboses or obstetric morbidity require monitoring during each pregnancy to ensure that the risk of further complications is reduced. Pre-conception, they should be tested for anti-Ro antibodies due to their association with the development of congenital foetal heart block (2% risk) and neonatal lupus (10% risk), which is discussed further in Chapters 1, 2.5, and 6. They should also be counselled for monitoring for symptoms of VTE and stroke with early presentation for assessment—there is 10-fold increased total risk of thrombosis in pregnancy for women with APS compared with those without, with a 6.5-fold increase in risk of stroke and 5–8-fold risk of VTE. They should also be advised not to become pregnant if there is a recent thrombosis within the last 3 months or uncontrolled hypertension. Medications should also be reviewed prior to conception or if not, early in pregnancy. Hydroxychloroquine, low-dose prednisolone, low-dose aspirin, azathioprine, and LMWH can be used safely in pregnancy (see also Chapters 3.1 and 3.2) in these patients.

During pregnancy, the best predictor of outcome is the previous pregnancy. Those with a poor obstetric history or who are primigravida should have regular foetal monitoring to assess for foetal growth restriction and pre-eclampsia. At each antenatal appointment, women should have urinalysis for proteinuria and blood pressure monitoring to screen for pre-eclampsia. In our unit, uterine artery Doppler velocimetry is performed in the 2nd trimester with detailed anatomy scans to assess for uterine arterial notching between 20–24 weeks as it has prognostic significance in APS pregnancies. Bilateral notching at week 20–24 is associated with the development of pre-eclampsia with sensitivity of 19% and specificity of 99%, indicating women who are at high risk requiring further monitoring.

Anticoagulation for those with antiphospholipid antibodies or antiphospholipid syndrome in pregnancy

Women with persistent aPL or APS should be started on low-dose aspirin (LDA) with/without LMWH when becoming pregnant. The use of LMWH is dependent upon their previous thrombotic and obstetric history shown in Table 2.1.3. Typically, higher doses of anticoagulation are used in women with arterial events than those with one-off VTE.

Heparin intolerance during pregnancy

Women who have intolerance to LMWH should be treated with a different formulation of LMWH initially. If there is no improvement with switching formulations, fondaparinux (a pentasaccharide with anti-Xa activity) or danaparoid can be used instead although their safety in pregnancy is less well described. There is a theoretical possibility they may be less efficacious in APS as they lack the anti-complement activity that heparins possess.

Heparin-induced thrombocytopenia (HIT) is a prothrombotic condition caused by antibodies to heparin-PF4 complexes resulting in subsequent platelet activation and consumption. It can present with acute systemic reactions on administration of heparin and the development of new thromboses or necrotic skin lesions during heparin use typically 5–10 days after starting. Therefore, platelet counts should be assessed for the presence of thrombocytopenia in these situations. Although an

Table 2.1.3 Suggested antithrombotic therapy for APS in pregnancy (5)

Scenario	Treatment
Women with aPL but no clinical features of APS, or women with aPL and <3 early miscarriages	Pregnancy: LDA 75–100 mg Puerperium: prophylactic LMWH for 7 days*
Women with ≥3 consecutive early miscarriages but no thrombotic events	Pregnancy: LDA +/- prophylactic LMWH (stop at 14–20 weeks if uterine artery Doppler normal) Puerperium: prophylactic LMWH for 7 days*
Women with previous intrauterine growth restriction, pre-eclampsia before 32 weeks, or intrauterine death	Pregnancy: LDA and prophylactic LMWH Puerperium: prophylactic LMWH for 7 days*
Women with previous VTE, i.e. thrombotic APS and treated with VKA	Pregnancy: LDA and intermediate dose LMWH Puerperium: switch to VKA if previous unprovoked events 6 weeks LMWH if previous provoked events and stop
Women with previous arterial events and APS	Pregnancy: LDA—and intermediate dose LMWH Puerperium: prophylactic LMWH followed by VKA
Women with APS with acute thrombotic event during pregnancy (provoked event)	Pregnancy: LDA and high-dose LMWH Puerperium: continue LMWH or switch to VKA for 6 weeks with a minimum of 3 months of anticoagulation in full Anticoagulation should then be stopped

*10 days according to RCOG guidance. LDA—low-dose aspirin; LMWH—low-molecular-weight heparin; VKA—vitamin K antagonist.

immune-mediated process, HIT has not been described during pregnancy. There is therefore no advice to monitor platelet counts in pregnancy any more frequently in those receiving heparin.

Case 3: SLE and thrombotic APS with thrombotic complications postpartum

A 24-year-old patient became pregnant with a diagnosis of SLE, pernicious anaemia, previous PE, and extensive DVT that occurred at age 14. She was identified as having APS with triple positive aPL testing (lupus anticoagulant positive, IgG anticardiolipin antibody 31 U/L, and anti-beta-2-glycoprotein antibody 62 U/L). As a teenager she was poorly compliant with warfarin, had further DVTs, and developed post-thrombotic syndrome. She underwent venous stenting with a good clinical response a year previously. Prior to this pregnancy, she had three consecutive spontaneous miscarriages in the 1st trimester and no live births. Her routine management prior to pregnancy was with azathioprine, hydroxychloroquine, hydroxocobalamin injections, and warfarin with target INR 3–4. Upon diagnosis of pregnancy, warfarin was replaced with LMWH at treatment doses and her other medications were continued unchanged.

During early pregnancy, she had features of small joint arthralgia; uterine artery Doppler velocimetry performed at 20 weeks' gestation showed an increased pressure of 1.6 in both arteries, so she had increased monitoring for pre-eclampsia.

She presented at 29 weeks' gestation with lethargy, increased joint pain, a malar rash, and vasculitic skin lesions. She was given an intermediate dose of steroids (prednisolone 20 mg) for a flare of SLE, with symptomatic improvement. She had a spontaneous vaginal delivery at 37 weeks. She developed a postpartum haemorrhage (PPH) of 750 ml estimated blood loss and a large vulvar haematoma 2 days following delivery, which required cessation of anticoagulation and surgical decompression. Over the next few days, she was given dalteparin 5,000 units once daily, developed abdominal pain with CT showing splenic and renal infarcts. She restarted high-intensity anticoagulation with intravenous UFH and was then changed to warfarin with a target INR of 3–4. There were no further thrombotic or bleeding issues and her renal function improved steadily over the next few months.

Case discussion

This case highlights the management of a woman with thrombotic and obstetric APS complicated by PPH and thrombotic events in the postpartum period.

Thrombosis recurrence with antiphospholipid syndrome during pregnancy

As discussed previously in case 2, thrombosis recurrence is a risk in pregnancy in APS and therefore clinicians must have a low threshold for further diagnostic imaging as discussed in case 1 for venous thromboses. An interesting feature of APS is that recurrent events typically occur in the same vascular bed causing similar patterns of thrombosis. Those with arterial thrombosis are more likely to have arterial thrombotic recurrence than those with VTE. Recurrence is more likely to occur at times of added prothrombotic risks such as acute illness, pregnancy, and surgery.

Women with APS with cerebral events have a 5% risk of recurrent neurological events during pregnancy. Those presenting with features of stroke should undergo imaging to clarify the cause including an ischaemic event, haemorrhage, particularly for those on anticoagulation or with a history of venous sinus thrombosis, of which the latter are most frequently seen in the 1st trimester. Magnetic resonance imaging (MRI) is preferable due to the risk of radiation exposure with CT as well as providing a more detailed view of cerebral parenchymal damage and vessel abnormalities.

Anticoagulation should be reviewed if further thrombotic events occur including assessment for compliance and anti-Xa monitoring particularly in those with extremes of weight. Dose increments of LMWH are required for those with further events. Women may need intravenous UFH peri-delivery and is the preferred initial anticoagulant in patients with haemodynamic instability as a result of large volume PE.

Catastrophic APS (CAPS) is the development of concurrent ≥3 organ thromboses within days, with the presence of antiphospholipid antibodies in serum and presence of thrombosis on organ histology. The mortality of CAPS is 30–50% and treatment is based upon high-intensity anticoagulation, plasma exchange (PEX), and intravenous immunoglobulins. The woman discussed in this case did not fulfil this diagnosis as fewer than three vascular sites were involved. However, CAPS should be considered early as part of the differential diagnosis given the sequential nature of her thromboses, multiple sites affected, and given the poor prognosis associated with the syndrome. Given the development of new thrombotic events, this patient should receive high-dose anticoagulation but further treatment such as PEX is not necessary unless further organs are thrombosed.

Adjuvants to treatment of antiphospholipid syndrome in pregnancy

The current mainstay of management for APS in pregnancy is LDA and LMWH, which achieves live pregnancies in 80%. Unfortunately, there remain 20% who still have pregnancy losses so additional treatments need to be considered. There is increasing data in small case series for those with recurrent thromboses or adverse obstetric outcomes with low-dose steroids and statins. Outcomes of large randomized controlled studies for added hydroxychloroquine are awaited. Currently, they are not recommended as up-front treatment of APS but can be considered in patients with refractory disease. Outside of pregnancy, increased thrombotic rates have been seen with the use of DOACs, particularly in patients with triple-positive APS, and there has been a European Medicines Agency alert advising DOACs should not be used in APS particularly in those who are triple positive.

Hydroxychloroquine is an antimalarial that has been extensively utilized for its anti-inflammatory properties to control systemic symptoms in SLE during pregnancy. There is evidence that there is an improvement in obstetric outcomes in women with APS, along with aspirin, and LMWH in those who are refractory to these treatments. There is also a suggestion that it can be used to decrease the thrombotic risk in patients with persistent aPL and APS in combination with anticoagulation. This may be due to its ability to inhibit aPL binding to endothelium and trophoblasts, maintaining the anticoagulant annexin-A5 shield of phospholipid membranes, and reducing platelet activation and aggregation.

Statins inhibit the hepatic enzyme HMG-CoA reductase and are used to lower systemic cholesterol levels particularly in patients with atherosclerotic disease. They have also been found to have multiple off-target anti-inflammatory and anticoagulant actions including a reduction in interleukin-6 (IL-6), vascular endothelial growth factor (VEGF), tumour necrosis factor α (TNF-α) levels, and lower expression of tissue factor. A small case series has shown an improvement in placental blood flow and a reduction in premature births with pravastatin in combination with aspirin and LMWH. The use of fluvastatin has shown lower levels of pro-inflammatory molecules in patients with antiphospholipid antibodies.

Low-dose steroids (prednisolone 10 mg) can be used in patients with APS with recurrent early pregnancy losses in combination with low-dose aspirin and LMWH in the 1st trimester.

There are to date no randomized controlled trials to inform on the use of statins, steroids, or hydroxychloroquine to improve pregnancy outcomes in women with APS. However, a currently ongoing RCT on hydroxychloroquine in pregnant women with aPL will hopefully provide the answer whether its use in addition to standard of care reduces pregnancy morbidity in these women.

Key messages

- Women with rheumatic diseases have a significantly increased risk of thrombosis during pregnancy and thromboprophylaxis should be considered on a case-by-case basis during pregnancy and the postpartum period.
- The development of VTE is the main direct cause of maternal death and its diagnostic and treatment approach is different to that in non-pregnant patients.
- The management of anticoagulation during pregnancy, delivery, and the puerperium requires experience and each case should be reviewed for thrombotic and bleeding risk factors throughout this period.
- APS should be considered as a diagnosis in women with autoimmune diseases who have thromboses or pregnancy-related complications or losses.
- The management of APS during pregnancy is typically complex requiring increased maternal and foetal monitoring with low-dose aspirin and LMWH as the mainstay of treatment. Additional drugs are currently being evaluated to reduce thrombosis and pregnancy losses and can be considered in refractory cases.

Further reading

1. https://www.npeu.ox.ac.uk/mbrrace-uk/reports/confidential-enquiry-into-maternal-deaths [Accessed 31st May 2019].
2. https://www.rcog.org.uk/en/guidelines-research-services/guidelines/gtg37a/ [Accessed 31st May 2019].
3. Goodacre S, Horspool K, Shephard N, et al. Selecting pregnant or postpartum women with suspected pulmonary embolism for diagnostic imaging: The DiPEP diagnostic study with decision-analysis modelling. *Health Technol Assess.* 2018;22(47):1–230.
4. National Institute for Health and Care Excellence. Venous thromboembolic diseases: Diagnosis, management and thrombophilia testing. *NICE Guidelines* [NG158]. 2020.
5. Schreiber K, Sciascia S, de Groot PG, et al. Antiphospholipid syndrome. *Nat Rev Dis Primers.* 2018;4:17103.
6. van der Pol LM, Tromeur C, Bistervels IM, et al. Pregnancy-adapted YEARS algorithm for diagnosis of suspected pulmonary embolism. *NEJM.* 2019;380:1139–49.
7. Righini M, Robert-Ebadi H, Elias A, et al. diagnosis of pulmonary embolism during pregnancy: A multicenter prospective management outcome study. *Ann Int Med.* 2018;169(11):766–73.

2.2

Prevention of postpartum venous thromboembolism (VTE)

Roseann O'Doherty and Fionnuala Ní Ainle

Introduction

Venous thromboembolism (VTE) is a major cause of maternal death in pregnancy and the postpartum period. Moreover, maternal morbidity associated with VTE can result in lifelong disability and psychological consequences (1, 2). VTE risk rises during pregnancy and peaks in the postpartum period (3).

Risk factors for postpartum VTE

The baseline pregnancy-associated VTE (PA-VTE) risk is further increased by additional maternal, pregnancy, and delivery characteristics. These have mainly been identified in registry studies or case-control studies. In a recently published cross-sectional study from 21,019 sequential postpartum VTE risk assessments, over three-quarters of women had at least one VTE risk factor and over 40% had two or more (4). Critically, in 19% of women, all VTE risk developed during delivery or in the postpartum period (not present prior to this peripartum period), *highlighting the importance of performing VTE risk assessment not only in early pregnancy but also after delivery.*

An interesting insight into the interaction of postpartum risk factors was provided by a large hospital-based case-control study in which VTE risk factors were validated by review of medical records, including 559 women with objectively verified VTE during pregnancy or the postpartum period and 1,229 controls (5). Risk factors for postnatal VTE included: antepartum immobilization, intrauterine growth restriction (IUGR), pre-eclampsia, emergency (but not elective) Caesarean section (CS), and postpartum haemorrhage (PPH). Some risk factors exhibited additive interaction while others appeared to act as multipliers. For example, antepartum immobilization with a high body mass index (BMI) and PPH necessitating reoperation for bleeding exhibited apparent multiplicative effects on the risk of postpartum VTE.

A risk prediction model for postpartum VTE was recently developed: emergency CS, stillbirth, varicose veins, pre-eclampsia/eclampsia, infection, and medical comorbidities were the strongest VTE predictors in the final model. The risk prediction model was able to discriminate postpartum women with and without VTE, with excellent calibration of observed versus the predicted VTE risks (6).

Caesarean section (CS)

The reported increased incidence associated with CS varies between studies. Risks appear higher following emergency CS (3). Consequently, recent consensus guidelines recommend thromboprophylaxis after emergency CS but not after elective CS if no other risk factors are present (7, 8).

Pre-eclampsia

Pre-eclampsia is characterized by maternal hypertension and proteinuria developing after 20 weeks' gestation and complicates up to 7% of pregnancies (9). Maternal coagulation and platelet activation occur during the systemic phase of this disorder. Pre-eclampsia increases the risk of postnatal VTE (10), with an up to 5-fold elevated risk when there is associated IUGR (5).

Infection

Infection is a procoagulant state and is well-established to be associated with an increased VTE risk in the non-pregnant patient (9). A recent study specifically investigated the effect of co-existing infection on VTE risk, and reported a 20- and 6-fold increased risk after vaginal delivery and CS respectively (5).

Haemorrhage

Several studies report a significant increase in PA-VTE risk in the setting of haemorrhage and blood transfusion (5, 9). PPH is associated with an up to 9-fold increased PA-VTE risk overall (9). A recent cohort study analysing this risk in more detail reported a 4-fold risk with a PPH >1000 ml not requiring surgical intervention, rising to 12-fold when surgical intervention for bleeding is required for the same bleed volume (5). Blood transfusion is also an independent major risk factor for both antenatal and postnatal VTE (5–7-fold increased risk) (9).

Obesity/elevated BMI

Obesity is associated with an elevated VTE risk both in the non-pregnant patient and during pregnancy and the puerperium (9). A Danish group specifically sought to assess the association of obesity (BMI >30) along with smoking on PA-VTE risk. Obesity was associated with an elevated VTE risk overall. Subsequent studies specifically addressing *antenatal* VTE risk associated with a BMI ≥25–30 have yielded widely varied results (0–9-fold elevated risk (9)) unless immobilized (the latter conferring a 62-fold elevated risk in one well-conducted study (5)). These same studies, when addressing *postnatal* VTE risk in patients with a BMI ≥25–30, have more consistently reported an increased VTE risk (approximately 2–5-fold) (9).

Prior VTE

Women with a personal VTE history have a higher risk of recurrent VTE during pregnancy (3). The absolute reported recurrence risk *appears highest for women with an unprovoked or a hormone-provoked VTE* while the VTE recurrence risk is much lower if the event was provoked by a major transient non-hormonal VTE risk factor (3).

Inherited thrombophilia

VTE risk is higher in pregnant women with inherited and acquired thrombophilia, particularly if associated with a family history of VTE. The reported increase in VTE risk varies widely depending on the type of thrombophilia (3).

Antiphospholipid syndrome (APS) and rheumatic conditions

APS is associated with an elevated VTE risk both in non-pregnant (11) and pregnant individuals, a 15-fold increase in PA-VTE risk having been reported in association with the latter (10). There is a dearth of high-quality data to support optimal management of these women with APS in the postpartum period, especially if there is prior history of VTE, when care plans should ideally be developed in collaboration with an experienced multidisciplinary team including a haematologist. However, the absolute risk of VTE in patients with purely obstetrical APS, with no prior VTE history, appears to be lower (~2-fold elevated risk (12)). Persistent antiphospholipid antibodies in connective tissue disorders and rheumatological conditions in the absence of a prior history of VTE appear to carry only a small additive risk for pregnancy complications (13). Recognizing the potential risk and individualizing VTE prevention strategies is critical.

Reducing the risk of VTE in pregnancy

For many VTE risk factors, the evidence base supporting optimal strategies for reducing the risk of postpartum VTE is weak. Indeed, the authors of a 2014 Cochrane review stated: 'there is insufficient evidence on which to base recommendations for thromboprophylaxis during pregnancy (*and that*) large scale, high-quality randomized trials of currently used interventions are warranted' (3). For women with prior VTE, it appears that this risk may be reduced by up to 75% with LMWH: studies evaluating LMWH during the antepartum and postpartum periods in women with prior VTE reported antepartum recurrence risks of 0.9% (95% CI 0.5–1.8%) with LMWH and 4.2% (95% CI 0.3–6.0%) without LMWH and postpartum recurrence risks of 1.7% (95% CI 1.2–2.7%) with LMWH and 6.5% (95% CI 4.3–9.7%) without LMWH (3). Current guidelines recommend that all pregnant women with a history of VTE should receive postpartum pharmacological thromboprophylaxis with LMWH, but that women with prior VTE that is either unprovoked or provoked by oestrogen or pregnancy should receive both antepartum and postpartum thromboprophylaxis (3, 7, 8, 14, Figure 2.2.1).

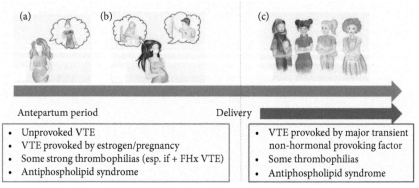

AREA OF UNCERTAINTY: multiple "common" risk factors
Interim solution: individualized risk assessment, shared decision-making?

Figure 2.2.1 Prevention of VTE in women with prior VTE or thrombophilia. FHx: family history

Guideline recommendations for PA-VTE risk reduction in women with inherited thrombophilia vary (7, 8, 14, 15). However, overall, guidelines suggest ante- and post-partum thromboprophylaxis in pregnant women with 'high-risk' thrombophilias especially when accompanied by a strong family history (Figure 2.2.1), but not for 'low-risk' thrombophilias (for which either postpartum thromboprophylaxis only or no thromboprophylaxis may be recommended).

For women with APS, there is no randomized trial data to support recommendations for optimal thromboprophylactic strategies in pregnancy. UK guidelines recommend that women with APS and a history of VTE (who will often be on long-term oral anticoagulation) should be offered thromboprophylaxis with LMWH (either 50%, 75%, or full treatment dose) antenatally and for 6 weeks postpartum or until returned to oral anticoagulant therapy after delivery (7). For women with antiphospholipid antibodies in connective tissue or rheumatic conditions but no history of prior VTE, another position paper suggests that thromboprophylaxis only be considered if additional risk factors are present and that any woman receiving antenatal LMWH should continue this for 6 weeks postpartum (16).

Although probably the best quality data surrounding VTE risk reduction address personal VTE history or inherited thrombophilia, these are rare (<1% in a recent large prospective study (4)). VTE prevention in women with more common VTE risk factors is a knowledge gap in 2020, as evidenced by widely varying international guideline recommendations (3, 7, 8, 14, 15). In a recent analysis of data from 21,019 consecutive comprehensive postpartum VTE risk assessments, applying the recommendations of representative international guidelines and calculating the proportion of women who would have received a recommendation for postpartum thromboprophylaxis under each guideline (4), this proportion ranged from 7% under American College of Obstetricians and Gynecologists (ACOG) guidelines (15) to 37% under UK Royal College of Obstetricians and Gynecologists (RCOG) guidelines (7).

Several international groups are prioritizing this research question: for example, in a recent multicentre study, vascular events occurred in 190 (19.2%) women before and 140 (13%) after implementation of risk score-driven prophylaxis (relative risk [RR] 0.68 [0.55; 0.83] and the incidence of pregnancy-associated DVT (PA-DVT) was reduced (RR 0.30 [0.14; 0.67]). PPH was recorded in 3.2% of women before and 4.5% after implementation (RR 1.38 [0.89; 2.13], p = 0.15).

Conclusions

International guidelines differ in recommendations on optimal management of 'common' VTE risk factors and duration of postpartum thromboprophylaxis (Figure 2.2.1). There is little available evidence to guide management and each option has potential risks and benefits. This important area remains a key knowledge gap in need of urgent high-quality evidence. However, there is little debate surrounding the requirement to perform systematic VTE risk assessment in pregnant and postpartum women: in a recent review of international guidelines, eight of nine recommended that all women should also undergo VTE risk-factor assessment (17). Recognizing the potential risk and individualizing VTE prevention strategies is critical. Risk factors commonly arise for the first time in the postpartum period (4). Performing postpartum systematic VTE risk assessment can be incredibly challenging. However, when this complex, multi-step process is streamlined, risk assessment of a very high proportion of women is feasible (18).

Guideline recommendations around VTE and thrombophilia can be broadly summarized as follows: antenatal and postnatal thromboprophylaxis is recommended for women with prior unprovoked VTE or VTE provoked by oestrogen or pregnancy (Figure 2.2.1 (a)), and for some strong thrombophilias, particularly if associated with a family history of VTE (Figure 2.2.1 (b)), due to a higher predicted recurrence risk than for women with a VTE provoked by a major transient non-hormonal provoking factor and some weaker thrombophilias, for whom only postnatal thromboprophylaxis is recommended (Figure 2.2.1 (c)).

Key messages

- VTE is a leading cause of death and morbidity in pregnant and postpartum women.
- Additional risk factors (including rheumatic disorders) may increase this risk.
- VTE risk assessment and implementation of appropriate thromboprophylaxis is essential in this population.
- Evidence gaps should be urgently addressed as research priorities.

Further reading

1. Konstantinides SV, Meyer G, Becattini C, et al. ESC Guidelines for the diagnosis and management of acute pulmonary embolism developed in collaboration with the European Respiratory Society (ERS). *Eur Heart J.* 2020 Jan 21;41(4):543–603. doi: 10.1093/eurheartj/ehz405.

2. de Wit K. Addressing emotional and physical distress after pulmonary embolism. *Thromb Res.* 2019. doi: 10.1016/j.thromres.2019.07.025 [published Online First: 2019/08/11].
3. Ewins K, Ní Áinle F. VTE risk assessment in pregnancy. *Res Pract Thromb Haemost.* 2020 (in press). Doi: org/10.1002/rth2.12290.
4. O'Shaughnessy F, Donnelly JC, Bennett K, et al. Prevalence of postpartum venous thromboembolism risk factors in an Irish urban obstetric population. *J Thromb Haemost.* 2019 Nov;17(11):1875–85. doi: 10.1111/jth.14568 [published Online First: 2019/07/17].
5. Jacobsen AF, Skjeldestad FE, Sandset PM. Ante- and postnatal risk factors of venous thrombosis: A hospital-based case-control study. *J Thromb Haemost.* 2008;6(6):905–12. doi: 10.1111/j.1538-7836.2008.02961.x.
6. Sultan AA, West J, Grainge MJ, et al. Development and validation of risk prediction model for venous thromboembolism in postpartum women: Multinational cohort study. *BMJ.* 2016;355:i6253. doi: 10.1136/bmj.i6253.
7. Reducing the risk of venous thromboembolism during pregnancy and the puerperium. *Royal College of Obstetricians and Gynaecologists Green-top Guideline No 37a.* 2015. See https://www.rcog.org.uk/globalassets/documents/guidelines/gtg-37a.pdf.
8. Bates SM, Greer IA, Middeldorp S, et al. VTE, thrombophilia, antithrombotic therapy, and pregnancy: Antithrombotic therapy and prevention of thrombosis, 9th ed: American College of Chest Physicians evidence-based clinical practice guidelines. *Chest.* 2012;141(2 Suppl):e691S–736S. doi: 10.1378/chest.11-2300.
9. Kevane B, Donnelly J, D'Alton M, et al. Risk factors for pregnancy-associated venous thromboembolism: A review. *J Perinat Med.* 2014;42(4):417–25. doi: 10.1515/jpm-2013-0207.
10. James AH, Jamison MG, Brancazio LR, et al. Venous thromboembolism during pregnancy and the postpartum period: Incidence, risk factors, and mortality. *Am J Obstet Gynecol.* 2006;194(5):1311–15. doi: S0002-9378(05)02452-X [pii] 10.1016/j.ajog.2005.11.008 [published Online First: 2006/05/02].
11. Keeling D, Mackie I, Moore GW, et al. Guidelines on the investigation and management of antiphospholipid syndrome. *Br J Haematol.* 2012;157(1):47–58. doi: 10.1111/j.1365-2141.2012.09037.x.
12. Gris JC, Bouvier S, Molinari N, et al. Comparative incidence of a first thrombotic event in purely obstetric antiphospholipid syndrome with pregnancy loss: The NOH-APS observational study. *Blood.* 2012;119(11):2624–32. doi: 10.1182/blood-2011-09-381913.
13. Soh MC, Pasupathy D, Gray G, et al. Persistent antiphospholipid antibodies do not contribute to adverse pregnancy outcomes. *Rheumatology.* 2013;52(9):1642–7. doi: 10.1093/rheumatology/ket173.
14. Bates SM, Rajasekhar A, Middeldorp S, et al. American Society of Hematology 2018 guidelines for management of venous thromboembolism: Venous thromboembolism in the context of pregnancy. *Blood Adv.* 2018;2(22):3317–59. doi: 10.1182/bloodadvances.2018024802.
15. James A, Birsner M, Kaimal A, et al. ACOG Practice Bulletin No. 196: Thromboembolism in Pregnancy. *Obstet Gynecol.* 2018;132(1):e1–e17. doi: 10.1097/aog.0000000000002706 [published Online First: 2018/06/26].
16. Knight CL, Nelson-Piercy C. Management of systemic lupus erythematosus during pregnancy: Challenges and solutions. *Open Access Rheumat.* 2017;9:37–53. doi: 10.2147/OARRR.S87828.
17. Okoroh EM, Azonobi IC, Grosse SD, et al. Prevention of venous thromboembolism in pregnancy: A review of guidelines, 2000–2011. *J Womens Health* (Larchmt). 2012;21(6):611–15. doi: 10.1089/jwh.2012.3600 [published Online First: 2012/05/05].
18. O'Shaughnessy F, Donnelly JC, Cooley SM, et al. Thrombocalc: Implementation and uptake of personalized postpartum venous thromboembolism risk assessment in a high-throughput obstetric environment. *Acta Obstet Gyn Scan.* 2017;96:1382–90. doi: 10.1111/aogs.13206.

2.3

Pulmonary arterial hypertension

Eliza Chakravarty

Introduction

Pulmonary arterial hypertension (PAH) can arise from many causes, including congenital heart disease, valvular heart disease, obesity, systemic hypertension, in addition to primary PAH and connective tissue disease-associated PAH (CTD-PAH). Although most of the principles outlined in this chapter will apply to all women with or at risk for PAH, the main focus will be on women with or suspected CTD-PAH. Normal, healthy pregnancy requires significant cardiopulmonary physiological changes to support the growing foetus. These include an increase in blood volume, cardiac output, basal oxygen consumption, and alveolar ventilation. Decreases in systemic and pulmonary vascular resistance help to accommodate those changes. However, in the setting of the non-inflammatory vasculopathy associated with CTD-PAH, the pulmonary vasculature is incapable of successfully accommodating the increased blood volume and increases pressure on the right ventricle.

Pre-conception counselling and risk stratification

Pre-conception PAH is associated with extremely elevated risks of morbidity and mortality for both mother and foetus. Maternal mortality rates for women with PAH are estimated to be between 8–16%, and death is often attributed to right heart failure. Delivery and the early postpartum period appear to be the most vulnerable for right heart failure and death. Women with known CTD-PAH should be strongly counselled against any future pregnancies and permanent or long-term reversible contraception strongly recommended. In addition, women with pre-existing PAH who become pregnant should consider termination of the pregnancy to protect the life of the mother. However, childbearing is extremely important for many women, and such pregnancies may be desired. In these cases, women should be counselled about the risks and monitored closely but should be supported in their decisions to proceed with their pregnancy in a non-judgemental manner. Wherever possible, treatment of PAH should be maximized with medications compatible with pregnancy prior to conception, including discontinuation of endothelin receptor antagonists and oral anticoagulants. Pregnancies should be managed with a specialized team of pulmonologists, rheumatologists, and maternal-foetal-medicine specialists.

Diagnosis during pregnancy

Case 1: Evaluation of a pregnant woman with dyspnea

A 27-year-old woman is 18 weeks into her first pregnancy. She has noted 2–3 weeks of progressive dyspnea and reduced exercise tolerance. She denies any chest pain, palpitations, lower extremity edema, or other symptoms, but is concerned that her dyspnea seems abnormal. Five years previously, she was found to have a positive antinuclear antibody (ANA) upon evaluation for a mild malar rash and Raynaud's phenomenon without digital ulcers; and she has been taking hydroxychloroquine since then without any further manifestations.

Case discussion

The evaluation of dyspnea in a pregnant woman can be a complicated issue as some mild degree of dyspnea can occur in even uncomplicated pregnancies as part of normal physiological changes of pregnancy. A mild dilutional anaemia combined with an increase of basal oxygen consumption by 50% and increase in alveolar ventilation that accompany a reduction in pulmonary vascular resistance. So, determining the degree of dyspnea that would trigger an evaluation is not completely clear. However, in this case of a young woman with some underlying autoimmune manifestations that are suggestive of lupus, it would not be unwarranted to proceed with an evaluation.

Because pregnancy is inherently a pro-thrombotic state and pulmonary emboli can be immediately life threatening, any evaluation of dyspnea should begin with an assessment of risk of venous thromboembolism (VTE). To further complicate the issue, D-dimer levels are often elevated in uncomplicated pregnancies and many imaging techniques used to diagnose VTE involve radiation to the chest and upper abdomen. Despite these caveats, it is critical to diagnose and initiate treatment if a PE is suspected, and it is equally important to eliminate PE as a cause of dyspnea to avoid unnecessary anticoagulation. Recently, an elegant algorithm has been published to diagnose pulmonary embolism in pregnant women (3) that was demonstrated to be effective in a study of 441 pregnant women. Importantly, no women for whom PE was excluded developed symptomatic VTE for the remainder of their pregnancy. Women with clinically suspected PE first underwent D-dimer testing. If the D-dimer was normal, PE was excluded. If D-dimer was positive, then women underwent bilateral leg compression ultrasound, with anticoagulation started if results showed evidence of VTE. Women with a negative ultrasound then underwent computed tomography pulmonary angiography (CTPA). Inconclusive results then led to ventilation/perfusion (V/Q) scan. Positive results were then treated with full anticoagulation using heparin with or without low-dose aspirin. A separate study evaluated a somewhat different algorithm that utilized both compression lower extremity US and D-dimer. If both were normal, VTE was excluded (5). The goal of these studies was to avoid exposure to radiation while maximizing sensitivity of diagnosis. However, the consequences of a missed and untreated VTE can be life threatening, so clinical suspicion should drive the decision to proceed with cardiopulmonary imaging even when D-dimer and/or compression ultrasounds are within normal limits.

Once VTE is excluded, the next important evaluation in a pregnant woman with a known or suspected underlying connective tissue disease should be for pulmonary arterial hypertension, as this is also a potentially life-threatening condition that requires immediate therapy, as women with PAH have a restricted capacity to handle the normal physiological increases in blood volume during pregnancy. Noninvasive testing for PAH includes echocardiogram with elevated pulmonary arterial pressure >30 mm Hg or pulmonary function tests showing an isolated reduction in diffusion capacity (DLCO), as assessed using carbon monoxide. In rare cases, right heart catheterization may be necessary. It is unclear if the normal parameters of these tests are altered due to pregnancy itself.

Management of PAH during pregnancy

Case 2: Pregnancy in a woman with known PAH

A 24-year-old woman with SLE was diagnosed with PAH 2 years earlier based upon right heart catheterization (pulmonary arterial pressure 55 mm Hg) now presented with an intrauterine pregnancy at 7 weeks' gestational age. Current medications were warfarin, sildenafil, hydroxychloroquine, ambresentin, and prednisone 15 mg daily. She had no evidence of congestive heart failure or any respiratory symptoms. After extensive counselling regarding the risks of continuing with pregnancy, she expressed a strong desire for the pregnancy and declined termination. Endothelin antagonist and warfarin were discontinued and full dose low-molecular-weight heparin was added to her regimen. At 17 weeks' gestation, she presented with fluid overload and was diagnosed with right heart failure. Furosemide and inhaled prostacyclin were added to manage PAH during 2nd trimester of pregnancy. She was admitted again at week 23 for exacerbation of congestive heart failure, at which time inhaled prostacyclin was discontinued and an intravenous prostacyclin pump was initiated. At 32 weeks, she underwent scheduled Caesarean delivery of an infant weighing 1750 grams, 1- and 5-minute appearance, pulse, grimace, activity, and respiration (APGAR) scores were 3 and 7 respectively. Bilateral tubal ligation was performed following delivery. The infant required a several-weeks admission to the neonatal intensive care unit, and the patient was admitted to the intensive care unit for 1 week to manage congestive heart failure.

Case discussion

In this setting, the patient had a pre-established diagnosis of severe PAH, but decided to proceed with her pregnancy. She required treatment with vasodilators known to be compatible with pregnancy, which included calcium channel blockers, phosphodiesterase type V inhibitors (sildenafil), and intravenous prostacyclins. Additional therapeutic interventions such as inhaled prostacyclins as well as diuretics can minimize fluid overload from progressive right heart failure.

The endothelin receptor antagonists should be avoided as a class in pregnant women with PAH based on rodent models suggesting embryolethality as well as a characteristic pattern of malformations including craniofacial, heart, and great vessel anomalies. Human antenatal exposure to this class of drugs is extremely limited at this time, but the US Food and Drug Administration has strongly recommended pregnancy testing before prescribing endothelin receptor antagonists and monthly during use. Women who are receiving such medications who wish to become pregnant, should discontinue them prior to conception and be assured of optimal disease control with compatible agents prior to conception. Fortunately, there are alternative therapies that are very effective to modulate moderate to severe PAH such as the prostacyclins, so that switching to these agents before conception is warranted.

Delivery and the first few postpartum weeks are the most dangerous for pregnant women with PAH when the risk of right heart collapse is highest due to acute and dramatic shifts of blood volume and pressure. For this reason, delivery should be carefully planned with labour induction or Caesarean delivery scheduled in advance to avoid spontaneous labour during times when specialized delivery teams may not be available. Risks exist with both vaginal and Caesarean delivery: Caesarean delivery is associated with more abrupt haemodynamic and blood volume changes, but avoids fluid and pressure shifts of prolonged labour. Conversely, vaginal delivery usually results in less blood loss and acute haemodynamic changes. Mode of delivery should be individualized based upon risks and benefits specific to each situation. Because this patient had suffered several exacerbations of congestive heart failure from PAH during the 2nd trimester, she underwent scheduled Caesarean delivery followed by intensive care admission for close monitoring of PAH and heart failure and to titrate intravenous prostacyclins. After a week in the intensive care unit, her cardiorespiratory condition stabilized; however, she remained hospitalized for nearly a month in order to maximize her condition with medications she could maintain as an outpatient.

Conclusions

PAH is a manifestation of connective tissue disease that carries with it an extremely high risk of maternal morbidity and mortality. In general, women diagnosed with CTD-PAH during the childbearing years should be strongly counselled regarding the extremely high risks associated with pregnancy and permanent or long-acting contraception offered. For women who desire to become or continue with an inadvertent pregnancy, PAH and resulting congestive heart failure need to be managed aggressively with combinations of calcium channel blockers, phosphodiesterase inhibitors, prostacyclins, diuretics, and heparins. Delivery and the first postpartum weeks are times of extremely high risk of right heart failure. Delivery should be scheduled to prevent spontaneous delivery, and patients will require intensive monitoring during and after delivery.

In women with underlying connective tissue diseases, progressive or abrupt dyspnea should warrant an evaluation for both VTE and PAH. Algorithms are available to assist with evaluation for VTE that minimizes risk of radiation exposure while maximizing diagnostic potential. Treatment should be geared to the underlying cause of cardiorespiratory pathology.

Key messages

- PAH is associated with significant risk of maternal morbidity and death, most commonly from right heart failure.
- Delivery and early postpartum periods carry the highest risks for maternal death.
- Women with pre-existing PAH should be strongly counselled against becoming pregnant, and should consider permanent or long-acting contraception.
- Evaluation of pregnant women with dyspnea should begin with diagnosis or exclusion of VTE, and anticoagulation with heparin initiated if VTE is discovered.
- Vasodilators are the mainstay of management of PAH during pregnancy, and endothelin receptor antagonists should be avoided based upon a characteristic embryopathy detected in rodent teratogenicity studies.

Further reading

1. Olsson KM, Channick R. Pregnany in pulmonary arterial hypertension. *Eur Respir Rev.* 2016;25:361–63.
2. Chakravarty EF. Vascular complications of systemic sclerosis during pregnancy. *Int J Rheumatol.* 2010;2010: pii: 287248. doi: 10.1155/2010/287248.
3. Righini M, Robert-Ebadi H, Elias A, et al. Diagnosis of pulmonary embolism during pregnancy: A multicenter prospective management outcome study. *Ann Int Med.* 2018;169:766–73.
4. Guglieminotti J, Landau R, Friedman AM, Li G. Pulmonary hypertension during pregnancy in New York State, 2003–2014. *Mater Child Health J.* 2019;23:277–84.
5. van der Pol LM, Tromeur C, Bistervels IM, et al. Pregnancy-adapted algorithm for diagnosis of suspected pulmonary embolism. *New Engl J Med.* 2019;380:1139–49.

2.4

Advanced renal disease/renal impairment

Hannah Blakey and Kate Bramham

Introduction

Successful pregnancy is possible for patients with chronic kidney disease (CKD) but the risks of adverse outcome (including pre-eclampsia (PET), pre-term birth, and low birth weight) increase incrementally with severity of renal impairment. Pregnancy in women with CKD secondary to rheumatological disease carries additional complexity, including the need for immunosuppressive medication, and risk of disease flare. Thorough pre-conception counselling and intensive monitoring throughout pregnancy by specialist renal and obstetric teams are therefore crucial in optimizing outcomes for mother and baby.

Investigating abnormal renal function in pregnancy

Case 1

A 29-year-old female was admitted to hospital at 18 weeks' gestation in her first pregnancy with fever and abnormal renal function (creatinine 115 µmol/L, no previous baseline for comparison). Blood pressure (BP) was normal (112/62 mm Hg) but urinalysis was positive for blood and protein (protein–creatinine ratio (PCR) 137 mg/mmol). Renal ultrasound appeared normal, but fever and acute kidney injury (AKI) persisted despite antibiotic treatment for presumed urinary tract infection.

Immunology tests revealed positive anti-nuclear antibody, double stranded DNA (dsDNA) antibody 73 kU/L, normal complement 3 and 4, positive Ro and La antibodies, and negative antiphospholipid antibodies. The decision was made to perform a renal biopsy, which showed active lupus nephritis (class IV-G(A)).

After careful discussion of all available treatment options, including therapeutic abortion which the patient declined, pulsed intravenous (IV) methylprednisolone was commenced. She was then treated with oral prednisolone (30 mg initially with reducing regime to a daily maintenance dose of 5 mg), hydroxychloroquine 200 mg once daily, and azathioprine 100 mg once daily for the remainder of the pregnancy. Renal function and proteinuria gradually improved back to normal levels. BP increased after 30 weeks of pregnancy, and she was commenced on labetalol 200 mg twice daily. She was seen regularly throughout pregnancy by renal and obstetric teams and delivered a healthy male born at 37 weeks after planned induction of labour.

Case discussion: Renal physiology in normal pregnancy

Glomerular hyperfiltration and a resulting fall in serum creatinine is seen from early pregnancy, peaking in the early-2nd trimester. Estimated glomerular filtration rate (GFR) equations under-estimate renal function in pregnancy and serial creatinine concentrations should be used instead. A serum creatinine above 75 μmol/L in pregnancy should be considered outside of the normal range and warrants further investigation. Gestational ranges of normal creatinine during pregnancy are dynamic (e.g. 8 weeks 95% CI: 50, 65 μmol/L; 20 weeks 95% CI: 45, 59 μmol/L; 38 weeks 50, 70 μmol/L) (1).

The kidneys increase in size in pregnancy by up to 10%, with a minimum normal bipolar length of 10 cm. Pregnancy-related hydronephrosis is common (right-sided in 85% of cases), secondary to a progesterone-mediated reduction in ureteric tone, and mechanical compression against the pelvic brim by the gravid uterus.

Investigating abnormal renal function in pregnancy

AKI in pregnancy is most common during the 3rd trimester, as a result of hypertensive disorders of pregnancy (including PET), sepsis, and puerperal complications including haemorrhage.

Earlier in pregnancy, routine antenatal urinalysis and BP monitoring may lead to the identification of previously unrecognized CKD. Raised urine protein–creatinine ratio (urine PCR) (>30 mg/mmol) or serum creatinine >75 μmol/L is suggestive of kidney disease, and further investigation by repeat serum creatinine, urinalysis, full blood count, and immunology testing (antinuclear antibody, complements 3 and 4, antineutrophil cytoplasmic antibody, dsDNA, and immunoglobulins) are indicated. Renal ultrasound should be performed (note physiological hydronephrosis of pregnancy is common and may be difficult to distinguish from pathological causes).

Classification of severity of CKD outside of pregnancy is made by assessment of GFR and quantification of urinary protein content (albumin–creatinine ratio)—see Table 2.4.1. The shading indicates the risk of progression of renal disease, morbidity, and mortality as proteinuria increases and GFR declines.

- *Pre-eclampsia (PET)*
  PET (see also Chapter 6) affects around 5% of all pregnancies and is characterized by new onset hypertension (BP >140/90 mmHg) and proteinuria (>300 mg/24 hrs), or other end organ compromise, after 20 weeks' gestation. Diagnosing PET can be difficult in patients with renal disease, many of whom already have pre-existing hypertension and proteinuria. Clinical correlation is required to differentiate PET from other causes of renal impairment: see Table 2.4.2.
- *Role of renal biopsy in pregnancy*
  Renal biopsy is technically difficult after 20–24 weeks' gestation and risks complications including bleeding and foetal compromise. This must be balanced against the benefits of histological diagnosis enabling targeted treatment and prognostication. In highly selected cases of undiagnosed progressive kidney disease, early onset nephrotic syndrome, or unexplained AKI (<26 weeks), renal biopsy should be considered.

Table 2.4.1 Classification of chronic kidney disease

Increasing risk →

			ACR categories (mg/mmol), description and range		
			<3 Normal to mildly increased	3–30 Moderately increased	>30 Severely increased
GFR categories (ml/ml/1.73m²), description and range			A1	A2	A3
>90	Normal and high	G1 ('CKD stage 1')			
60–89	Mild reduction	G2 ('CKD stage 2')			
45–59	Mild–moderate reduction	G3a ('CKD stage 3a')			
30–44	Moderate–severe reduction	G3b ('CKD stage 3b')			
15–29	Severe reduction	G4 ('CKD stage 4')			
<15	Kidney failure/end stage renal disease	G5 ('CKD stage 5')			

Increasing risk ↑

Key: ACR categories—albumin–creatinine ratio; CKD—chronic kidney disease; GFR—glomerular filtration rate.

Table 2.4.2 Differentiating between normal pregnancy, CKD, active lupus nephritis, and PET

Clinical features	Normal pregnancy	CKD	Active lupus nephritis	PET
Hypertension	No	Yes	Yes	Yes (>20 weeks)
Proteinuria	No/<300 mg/day	Yes	Yes	Yes
Haematuria	No	Yes	Yes	No
Rate of change in serum creatinine	Small increase 3rd trimester	No change (unless disease progression/AKI)	Moderate to rapid increase (days)	Rapid increase (hours/days)
Uterine artery Doppler at >24 weeks	Normal	Normal	Normal	Abnormal 'notching' sometimes Raised pressure index
Blood tests	↑ESR	↓eGFR prior to pregnancy	↓C3/C4 ↑dsDNA	↑AST/ALT ↓platelets ↑urate ↓PlGF ↑sFlt-1

Key: CKD: chronic kidney disease, PET: pre-eclampsia, ESR: erythrocyte sedimentation rate, eGFR: estimated glomerular filtration rate, C3/C4: complement protein 3 and 4, dsDNA: anti-double stranded DNA antibody, AST: aspartate aminotransferase, ALT: alanine aminotransferase, PlGF: placental growth factor, sFlt-1: soluble fms-like tyrosine kinase-1.

Management of lupus nephritis in pregnancy

Systemic lupus erythematosus (SLE) predominantly affects women of childbearing age and does not appear to adversely affect fertility. Patients with SLE are at increased risk of complications in pregnancy including PET, pre-term delivery, pregnancy loss, and SLE flare. Active SLE, lupus nephritis, chronic hypertension, and presence of lupus anticoagulant are all predictors of adverse pregnancy outcome.

- *Treatment of active lupus nephritis in pregnancy*
  Prompt treatment of active SLE and lupus nephritis in pregnancy is required to optimize maternal and foetal outcomes. In early pregnancy with severe SLE flare, discussion around therapeutic abortion may be necessary to allow optimal treatment of the maternal condition.

  Cyclophosphamide and mycophenolate mofetil (MMF) are both effective induction agents in the treatment of lupus nephritis (see Chapter 3.1). However, cyclophosphamide is associated with significant teratogenic and foetotoxic effects and should not be used in pregnancy or breastfeeding. MMF is associated with an embryopathy comprising cleft lip and palate, ear and cerebral abnormalities in up to 25% which may be difficult to detect on foetal ultrasound. It should not be given in pregnancy or in the 3 months prior to conception. Rituximab crosses the placenta and has been associated with neonatal B cell depletion, and should be considered in severe disease only if no other medication can effectively control active lupus nephritis. See Table 2.4.4 (case 2) for further information.

When pregnancy is continued, first line therapy is pulsed intravenous methylprednisolone followed by maintenance oral prednisolone (rapidly tapered dose as tolerated). Azathioprine (or tacrolimus) steroid-sparing immunosuppression is also given, in addition to hydroxychloroquine. All are safe to use in pregnancy and breastfeeding, although steroids and tacrolimus increase the risk of gestational diabetes and women should undergo oral glucose tolerance testing at 26 weeks' gestation.

- Anticoagulation
  Prophylactic dose low-molecular-weight heparin (LMWH) should be considered in the following scenarios:
  - Presence of significant proteinuria (PCR or ACR ≥200 mg/mmol) with consideration of additional risk factors (low serum albumin, maternal age, obesity, hypertension).
  - Previous history of venous thromboembolic disease.
  - History of significant pregnancy loss in the presence of antiphospholipid antibodies.

Clearance of LMWH may be reduced in patients with renal impairment. It is therefore recommended to monitor anti-Factor Xa levels for this cohort: blood samples should be taken 3–5 hours post dose, with a target therapeutic range of 0.5–1.0 units/ml.

- PET prophylaxis
  All women with lupus should be commenced on low-dose aspirin from the 1st trimester to reduce their risk of developing PET, unless otherwise contraindicated.

Pre-pregnancy counselling in chronic kidney disease

Case 2

A 26-year-old female attends pre-pregnancy counselling clinic. She was diagnosed with ANCA-associated vasculitis 2 years prior after presenting with epistaxis, haemoptysis, and AKI. Relevant investigations revealed haematuria, proteinuria, a high PR3 antibody titre, and renal biopsy confirmed granulomatosis with polyangiitis. She was treated with methylprednisolone and pulsed IV cyclophosphamide and has not had any vasculitic relapses since diagnosis.

Her most recent blood tests are as follows: creatinine 80 μmol/L, eGFR 77 ml/min / 1.73 m^2, Hb 118 g/L, ANCA pos 1:25, anti-PR3 7, anti-MPO <2. Urine ACR is 2.0 mg/mmol. Her current medication comprises azathioprine 100 mg once daily, prednisolone 5 mg once daily, and Cerazette once daily.

She wishes to become pregnant and would like to discuss what the risks of pregnancy might be for her and for her baby. She is also concerned about the impact of previous cyclophosphamide treatment on her fertility.

Pre-pregnancy counselling for patients with renal disease

Advances in medical care have led to an increasing prevalence of complex renal disease in women of childbearing age. Women with CKD are at increased risk of adverse maternal and foetal outcomes in pregnancy, although the risks of pregnancy will depend upon underlying disease aetiology and severity, rate of decline of renal function, prior obstetric history, and presence of additional risk factors. Pre-pregnancy counselling should be offered to allow informed decision making and to facilitate discussion and preparation for the complications that pregnancy may confer. Pre-pregnancy counselling should include discussion of the following:

- *Effect of CKD on pregnancy outcomes*
  When compared to healthy pregnant women without CKD, women with CKD have significantly increased risks of maternal and foetal complications (including PET, requirement for Caesarean section, pre-term delivery, low-birth-weight babies, requirement for neonatal intensive care (NICU), and neonatal death) (2, 3). Absolute rates vary between studies and there is limited data for women with more advanced CKD (stages 4 and 5), but in general, the risks increase incrementally as renal function declines. See Table 2.4.3.

Additional risk factors for adverse pregnancy outcome include chronic hypertension, pre-existing proteinuria, prior kidney transplant, and lupus nephritis; independently of CKD severity. However, even patients with CKD stage 1 without hypertension, proteinuria or systemic disease have an elevated risk of adverse outcome when compared to the general population (odds ratio (OR) 1.88, 95% CI 1.27–2.79) (3).

Table 2.4.3 Effect of CKD on pregnancy outcomes

Maternal/Foetal outcome	CKD stage 1 (n = 370)	CKD stage 2 (n = 87)	CKD stage 3 (n = 37)	CKD stage 4–5 (n = 10)	p-value
Caesarean section (%)	48.4	70.1	78.4	70.0	<0.001
Gestational age (Weeks + Days)	37.6 ± 2.6	35.7 ± 3.2	34.4 ± 2.4	32.6 ± 4.2	<0.001
Pre-term delivery (<37 Week) (%)	23.5	50.6	78.4	88.9	<0.001
Birth weight (g)	2966.5 ± 659	2484 ± 707	2226.3 ± 582	1639 ± 870	<0.001
Small-for-gestational-age <10%	13.3	17.9	18.9	50.0	0.02
Requirement for NICU (%)	10.3	27.6	44.4	70.0	<0.001
CKD stage shift (%)	7.6	12.6	16.2	20.0	0.12

Data extracted from 2015 Italian cohort study of pregnancy outcomes in patients with CKD (4), and recorded as a percentage or mean ± SD.

- *Effect of pregnancy on maternal renal function*
  Women with CKD stages 1 and 2 with low level proteinuria and absent or well-controlled hypertension appear to be at low risk of accelerated decline in GFR post-pregnancy (2). However, those women with more advanced renal impairment (pre-pregnancy GFR <40 μmol/L and proteinuria >1 g/day) are at substantially increased risk of accelerated renal decline both during and after pregnancy (3).
- *Timing of pregnancy*
  Women with relapsing and remitting renal disease, including lupus nephritis and ANCA-associated vasculitis, have more favourable outcomes when pregnancy is deferred until a period of disease quiescence (ideally 6 months).

  Those with rapidly progressive renal dysfunction or receiving renal replacement therapy are best advised to wait until after successful renal transplantation before attempting to conceive. Those with a slowly progressive disease course who may not require a kidney transplant for some time should plan pregnancy earlier whilst being of childbearing age.
- *Immunosuppression in pregnancy*

See Table 2.4.4 and Chapter 3.1 for overview of immunosuppressive agents and pregnancy advice.

Cyclophosphamide and fertility:
- Cyclophosphamide is frequently used in the induction treatment of rapidly progressive glomerulonephritis. It is teratogenic and foetotoxic and should not be used in pregnancy.
- Cyclophosphamide is associated with age-dependent and dose-dependent (cumulative lifetime dose) gonadotoxicity and may cause irreversible infertility in females. The use of short courses of pulsed cyclophosphamide is not commonly associated with sustained amenorrhoea in younger women (<32 years old), although the risk of impaired fertility should always be discussed when proposing treatment to women of childbearing age, and fertility preservation options offered.

Timing of rituximab:
- Long-term child outcomes following in utero rituximab exposure remain unknown. Rituximab crosses the placenta and may cause neonatal B cell depletion, particularly if given during the 2nd and 3rd trimesters. Treatment with rituximab during pregnancy may however be considered in severe or organ-threatening disease in the absence of other treatment options (ideally in the pre-conception or early pregnancy period).

Contraception
Contraception counselling should be offered to all women of childbearing age with CKD to mitigate the risks of unplanned pregnancy in this already high-risk cohort.

Progesterone-only contraceptives, including the progesterone-only pill, intra-uterine devices (IUDs) such as the Mirena coil, and subdermal implants are well tolerated, safe, and highly effective for women with CKD. The use of IUDs in immunosuppressed women does not appear to be associated with an increased risk of pelvic infection.

Table 2.4.4 Immunosuppression and safety in pregnancy

Medication	Evidence of teratogenicity?	Comments
Azathioprine	No—continue in pregnancy	Foetal myelosuppression unlikely if total dose <2 mg/kg and maternal white cell count maintained within normal range.
Ciclosporin	No—continue in pregnancy	May be associated with lower birth weight. Monitor pre-dose drug levels. Average 40% dose increase required antenatally.
Cyclophosphamide	Yes—congenital abnormalities of skull, ear, face, limb, and visceral organs. Increased risk of miscarriage.	Ensure effective contraception during and 3 months post treatment.
Hydroxychloroquine	No—continue in pregnancy	Withdrawal may precipitate lupus flare. May reduce risk of foetal congenital heart block in anti-Ro/SSA positive mothers.
Mycophenolate	Yes—up to 40% spontaneous miscarriage rate. Embryopathy: cleft lip and palate, ear, and cerebral abnormalities in 25% of exposed pregnancies. May be difficult to detect on foetal ultrasound.	Stop *at least 3 months* before planned conception to enable transfer to alternative therapy (usually azathioprine) and assessment of stability, before attempting conception. Risk of disease flare during this period must be discussed.
Prednisolone	No—continue in pregnancy (doses of <15 mg/day not associated with teratogenicity or neonatal adrenal suppression).	Increased risk of gestational diabetes → glucose tolerance test required at 26 weeks.
Rituximab	Unclear—limited data. Risk of neonatal B cell depletion if given in 2nd and 3rd trimesters. Long-term effects unknown.	If no alternative options. IgG antibody will not cross placenta until 16 weeks' gestation.
Tacrolimus	No—continue in pregnancy	Increased risk of gestational diabetes (2–10%) → glucose tolerance test at 26 weeks. Monitor pre-dose drug levels. Dose increase often required.

Oestrogen-containing contraceptives are associated with an increased risk of hypertension and venous thromboembolism. They are contraindicated in women with risk factors such as antiphospholipid antibody syndrome or nephrotic syndrome and are generally avoided in women with CKD in favour of safer progesterone-only preparations.

Antenatal management of patients with chronic kidney disease

Case 3

A 29-year-old female attends antenatal clinic at 12 weeks of pregnancy. She has a background of SLE and was previously treated for lupus nephritis which has been in remission for the last 2 years. Her current medication includes prednisolone 5 mg once daily, azathioprine 100 mg once daily (switched from mycophenolate 8 months ago), hydroxychloroquine 200 mg once daily and nifedipine 20 mg once daily (switched from ramipril after positive pregnancy test).

Blood tests show stable CKD stage 4 (creatinine 185 µmol/L, eGFR 28 ml/min/1.73 m^2) and normal soluble immunology (normal C3/4, dsDNA <20 kU/L). There is moderate proteinuria (PCR 72 mg/mmol). BP is 128/82 mm Hg.

She is commenced on low-dose aspirin from 12 weeks' gestation and seen monthly throughout pregnancy in a specialist renal-obstetric clinic. She is commenced on labetalol in addition to nifedipine from 24 weeks' gestation due to rising blood pressure. Creatinine and proteinuria rapidly increased at 36 weeks' gestation, and a diagnosis of PET is made. A Caesarean section delivery is performed due to foetal concerns (abnormal cardiotocography (CTG)).

At 1 year postpartum her renal function had declined further: creatinine 256, eGFR 18. She plans to have more children but is worried about the risks of future pregnancy given her advancing kidney impairment.

Hypertension in pregnancy

Chronic hypertension has been strongly associated with adverse pregnancy outcomes including PET (relative risk [RR] 7.7; 95% CI 5.7–10.1), pre-term delivery (RR 2.7; 95% CI 1.9–3.6), low birth weight (RR 2.7; 95% CI 1.9–3.8), NICU admission (RR 3.2; 95% CI 2.2–4.4), and perinatal death (RR 4.2; 95% CI 2.7–6.5) (3) (see also Chapter 6).

- *BP targets in pregnancy*
  Historic concerns exist linking over-zealous BP control during pregnancy with an increased risk of foetal growth restriction. However, the Control of Hypertension in Pregnancy Study (CHIPS) trial found that 'tight' BP control (diastolic BP <85 mmHg) was *not* associated with adverse pregnancy outcomes when compared with 'less tight' control (diastolic BP <100 mmHg) (5). There was, however, an increased risk of developing severe maternal hypertension in the less tightly controlled group.

  Current consensus recommends treating BP to a target of <140/90 mmHg for women with CKD with chronic hypertension in pregnancy. However, there remains a lack of data specific to CKD, and evidence-based BP targets for this group are yet to be established.

- *Antihypertensive medication*

Women with chronic hypertension should ideally be established pre-pregnancy on safe antihypertensive treatment, including labetalol, nifedipine, or methyldopa. In practice, methyldopa tends to be less well tolerated than labetalol or nifedipine and has been linked to an increased risk of postnatal depression, so should be avoided in breastfeeding women.

Angiotensin-converting enzyme inhibitors (ACEi) and angiotensin receptor blockers (ARB) are commonly used as first-line agents for patients with proteinuric CKD. They have been associated with oligohydramnios and neonatal renal failure and should not be used in the 2nd and 3rd trimesters but appear safe in the 1st trimester. Selected patients with a high risk of progressive proteinuria or renal decline may continue to take ACEi/ARB in the pregnancy-planning period provided they are carefully counselled to discontinue the medication following a positive pregnancy test and are able to test early for pregnancy.

Pre-eclampsia (PET)

- *Prophylaxis*

Women with CKD have a substantially increased risk of PET. Incidence ranges from 20–60% depending on the severity of pre-pregnancy renal dysfunction and presence of pre-existing proteinuria or hypertension.

Current guidelines recommend the use of low-dose aspirin (typically 75 mg daily) for all women considered to be at high risk of PET from 12 weeks' gestation until delivery. This includes all women with pre-existing renal disease (irrespective of CKD severity). Prophylactic treatment with aspirin has led to a reduced risk of developing PET and associated adverse pregnancy outcomes, with no evidence of increased risk of bleeding complications.

- *Diagnosis in CKD*

Many women with CKD have pre-existing hypertension and/or proteinuria, making the diagnosis of PET difficult. Discriminatory factors are listed in Table 2.4.2 (case 1). In practice, observing the progression of signs and symptoms over time is key; changes in proteinuria and BP tend to occur more rapidly in PET than in CKD. Anti-angiogenic/angiogenic biomarkers (soluble Fms-like tyrosine kinase receptor-1 (sFlt-1) and placental growth factor (PlGF)) appear to be promising adjuncts to diagnosis of PET in women with CKD (3).

- *Treatment*

Antenatal management of PET is focused on controlling BP and carefully observing mother and foetus for adverse signs (including regular CTG, growth scanning, and umbilical artery Doppler assessment) that may necessitate expedited delivery. Delivery of the foetus (and placenta) ultimately remains the only definitive treatment option.

Proteinuria in pregnancy

Women with CKD should be screened for proteinuria at every antenatal visit, with formal quantification using protein–creatinine or albumin–creatinine ratio (PCR or ACR).

Moderate proteinuria detected early in pregnancy frequently progresses to heavy proteinuria, sometimes into the nephrotic range in the 3rd trimester. Heavy proteinuria substantially increases the thromboembolic risk, and prophylactic dose LMWH is indicated in this setting. The threshold level of proteinuria for initiating treatment is unclear, although many centres treat when PCR exceeds 200 mg/mmol. Monitoring anti-factor Xa activity (3 hours post-LMWH) improves the safety of treatment in patients with renal impairment.

Progression of maternal renal disease

A pre-pregnancy GFR <40 μmol/L and proteinuria >1 g/day have been associated with an accelerated decline in renal function at 6 months postpartum. Forty-three per cent of women with moderate to severe pre-pregnancy CKD have a permanent decline in renal function after pregnancy. Around one in ten progress to end stage renal disease (ESRD) and require dialysis within 6 months postpartum (although data is based on small historical cohorts) (3).

Fertility in women treated with chronic dialysis is markedly reduced, and conception rates are low. Despite this, there has been a significant rise in the number of successful pregnancies reported in recent years. Conception rates and pregnancy outcomes for women who progress to dialysis during pregnancy are superior to those already established on dialysis prior to pregnancy.

Dialysis patients have high rates of maternal and foetal complications in pregnancy, including pre-term delivery, low birth weight, and PET. However, a more recent trend towards intensive daily dialysis regimes in pregnancy have led to improved outcomes. In a study comparing pregnancy outcomes of women receiving intensive haemodialysis (mean 43 hours per week) with patients receiving 'standard' dialysis (mean 17 hours per week), the intensive dialysis group had a significantly higher live birth rate (86.4% vs 61.4%, p = 0.03) and a longer median duration of pregnancy (36 weeks vs 27 weeks, p = 0.002) (3).

Fertility is rapidly restored following kidney transplantation, and pregnancy outcomes improve following successful transplantation when compared to women remaining on dialysis. Women requiring dialysis are therefore best advised to wait until after successful transplantation, if possible, before attempting to conceive.

Key messages

- CKD is associated with increased risks of adverse maternal and foetal pregnancy outcomes including PET, pre-term birth, and low birth weight. The risks increase incrementally with severity of CKD.

- Women with renal disease should be offered pre-conception counselling. Pregnancy planning should include substituting medications known to be teratogenic for safer alternatives and optimizing underlying disease control.
- Women with relapsing and remitting disease such as lupus and vasculitis should wait to conceive until a period of stability or disease quiescence for ≥6 months. Those with rapidly deteriorating renal function or already established on dialysis may have improved pregnancy outcomes by waiting until after successful kidney transplantation to conceive.
- All women with CKD should be offered low-dose aspirin from 12 weeks of pregnancy to reduce the risk of PET.

Further reading

1. Harel Z, McArthur E, Hladunewich M, Dirk JS, Wald R, Garg AX, et al. Serum creatinine levels before, during and after pregnancy. *JAMA*. 2019;321(2):205–7.
2. Zhang JJ, Ma XX, Hao L, Liu LJ, Lv JC, Zhang H. A systematic review and meta-analysis of outcomes of pregnancy in CKD and CKD outcomes in pregnancy. *Clin J Am Soc Nephrol*. 2015;10(11):1964–78.
3. Wiles KS, Nelson-Piercy C, Bramham K. Reproductive health and pregnancy in women with chronic kidney disease. *Nat Rev Nephrol*. 2018;14(3):165–84.
4. Piccoli GB, Cabiddu G, Attini R, Vigotti FN, Maxia S, Lepori N, et al. Risk of adverse pregnancy outcomes in women with CKD. *J Am Soc Nephrol*. 2015;26(8):2011–22.
5. Magee LA, von Dadelszen P, Rey E, Ross S, Asztalos E, Murphy KE, et al. Less-tight versus tight control of hypertension in pregnancy. *N Engl J Med*. 2015;372(5):407–17.

2.5

Antibodies as risk factors for adverse maternal and foetal outcomes

Massimo Radin, Karen Schreiber, and Savino Sciascia

Case 1: How to counsel a woman with persistent antiphospholipid antibodies (aPL) with no previous clinical manifestation who is planning a pregnancy through assisted reproduction

How to counsel a woman with persistent antiphospholipid antibodies (aPL) with no previous clinical manifestation who is planning a pregnancy through assisted reproduction.

A 21-year-old nurse presents in your clinic. As part of her work-up for IVF she has been found to be positive for lupus anticoagulant (LA). She has no pregnancy history and never had any thromboses in the past. She has no other past medical history, is normal weight with a body mass index (BMI) of 23, and she works in her spare time as a fitness instructor. You perform blood tests, and you confirm that she is positive for LA and a low titre of anticardiolipin (aCL) IgM antibodies. Her full blood count confirms a mild thrombocytopenia with platelets of $8^9 \times 10^9$/L. She would like to know your advice if this has implications for her IVF treatment.

Case discussion

Firstly, the patient can be reassured that she can undergo IVF despite being persistently positive for aPL. The available evidence on the efficacy and safety, of assisted reproduction techniques (ART), including ovulation induction therapy and IVF, in women with aPL stem from observational studies and recommendations regarding ART in women with aPL have been outlined in the European League against Rheumatism (EULAR) recommendations (1). Up to 30% achieve a pregnancy, which is comparable to the general population. ART are generally safe if the patient has quiescent disease and is on adequate thrombroprophylaxis or antithrombotic treatment depending on the aPL pattern or antiphospholipid syndrome (APS) clinical phenotype (thrombotic or obstetric APS) (1).

Although it is challenging to define a single protocol, some general measures for prophylaxis in aPL-positive women undergoing ovarian stimulation can be suggested. The type (low-dose aspirin (LDA), low molecular-weight heparin (LMWH)) and dosage (prophylactic versus full anticoagulant) of antithrombotic treatment should be recommended during pregnancy according to the individual risk profile (1).

In this case, the patient has not experienced any clinical manifestations of APS that fulfil the Sydney criteria. The general consensus is that, in pregnancy, these patients should receive LDA to reduce the risk of pre-eclampsia. Patients should also receive patient education and close monitoring during pregnancy. In case of IVF, LDA should be stopped three days before egg retrieval and resumed the following day. Patients with positive aPL who are not taking LDA during the ovarian stimulation period should start LDA on the day of the embryo transfer. All patients should also receive a thrombosis risk assessment according to local clinical guidelines to determine if a patient requires antenatal and postpartum LMWH. Please see Table 8.3.1 Chapter 8.3 for the management of women with aPL during pregnancy.

Overall, ovarian hyperstimulation syndrome can be avoided using milder hormonal stimulation or GnRH agonist protocols. The use of the 'natural cycle' method is another option, although it has a lower rate of pregnancy success rate. The ART induction protocol should be tailored to the individual patient, balancing the safety and effectiveness of the procedure.

In regard to her platelet counts, many patients with aPL have thrombocytopenia (platelets $<100 \times 10^9$/L). The pathogenic antibodies are directed towards platelet membrane glycoproteins and are distinct from aPL. Patients should be managed in the same way as for immune thrombocytopenia. In patients with a previous thrombosis, the fine balance between bleeding and thrombotic risk must be carefully managed and a platelet count $>50 \times 10^9$/L should be maintained to allow safe pharmacological thromboprophylaxis.

Case 2 : How to counsel a woman with aPL (triple positivity) and a previous single early miscarriage (<10 weeks) who is planning an IVF pregnancy

How to counsel a woman with aPL (triple positivity) and a previous single early miscarriage (<10 weeks) who is planning an IVF pregnancy.

A 25-year-old pharmacist presents in your APS pregnancy clinic. As part of her work-up for IVF she has been found to be positive for LA, aCL IgG antibodies, and beta2-glycoprotein1 (β2GPI) IgM antibodies. She had one previous single early miscarriage (<10 weeks) and never had any thromboses in the past. She has no other past medical history and has a BMI of 20. You perform blood tests, and you confirm that she is triple positive for aPL. She would like to know your advice going forward with her IVF treatment.

Case discussion

While the patient has a previous history of early miscarriage (<10 weeks), she does not fulfil the Sydney criteria for APS. The management of women with aPL who do not fulfil the obstetric or vascular criteria for definite APS is a matter of ongoing debate. In order to classify a patient as APS, according to the obstetric classification criteria, the number of previous early miscarriages should be three or more and these miscarriages should be consecutive. However, when clinical suspicion of APS is high, clinicians often start treatment in these women before the classification criteria are reached. Albeit the evidence is heterogeneous, LDA is often used (see Chapter 8.2) in these patients. Its use has been shown to reduce the risk of developing pre-eclampsia

---

Box 2.5.1 Definitions of medium-high antiphospholipid antibody (aPL) titres, and of high-risk and low-risk aPL profile (EULAR recommendations for the management of APS in adults 2019)

Medium-high aPL titres

Anticardiolipin (aCL) antibody of IgG and/or IgM isotype in serum or plasma present in titres >40 IgG phospholipid (GPL) units or >40 IgM phospholipid (MPL) units, or >the 99th percentile, measured by a standardized ELISA. Anti-beta2 glycoprotein I (anti-β2GPI) antibody of IgG and/or IgM isotype in serum or plasma in titre >the 99th percentile, measured by a standardized ELISA.

High-risk aPL profile

The presence (in 2 or more occasions at least 12 weeks apart) of lupus anticoagulant (measured according to International Society for Thrombosis and Haemostasis (ISTH) guidelines), or of double (any combination of lupus anticoagulant, aCL antibodies or antibeta2 glycoprotein I antibodies) or triple (all three subtypes) aPL positivity, or the presence of persistently high aPL titres.

Low-risk aPL profile

Isolated aCL or antibeta2 glycoprotein I antibodies at low/medium titres, particularly if transiently positive.

---

in high-risk patients, and the presence of aPL is a risk factor for the development of pre-eclampsia.

In general, the best predictor of maternal and foetal outcome in pregnancies in women with aPL is the previous obstetric history. With a previous normal obstetric history despite aPL, any future pregnancy is likely to have a low risk of complications and women can be reassured. Poor prognostic factors for pregnant women with aPL and APS include the presence of lupus anticoagulant (LA) and number of aPLs (Box 2.5.1). In prospective studies, LA appears to be the major predictor of poor pregnancy outcomes in the 2nd and 3rd trimester in women with aPL (2). The number of different aPL specificities also appears to be a poor prognostic factor. Retrospective multicentre data show that women with triple positive antibodies are at higher risk for pregnancy complications compared to women with single positivity (3).

Challenges in immunological testing

The detection and quantification of disease-associated biomarkers (mainly autoantibodies) is often central to a diagnosis, treatment, and monitoring of many autoimmune diseases. Early diagnosis, risk assessment, follow-up, and, in some cases, treatment are deeply influenced by immunological testing, especially when planning a pregnancy. The reliability of autoantibody measurements (= reproducibility of the test) and the diagnostic accuracy (= ability to identify patients at higher risk for a specific condition) are therefore crucial for optimum patient care and management.

Historically, qualitative or semi-quantitative indirect immunofluorescence assays have been used for the detection of autoantibodies. Enzyme-linked immunosorbent assay (ELISA)-based assays have been used as follow-up investigations to confirm and quantify the concentration of an autoantibody in blood serum. These measurements have traditionally been performed in specialized immunology laboratories. However, autoantibody testing is now commonplace with an increasing tendency towards more automated methods, in larger number of laboratories. As the number of testing increases, the number of available techniques for immunological testing is increasing as well. One of the main rising concerns of the treating clinician when prescribing immunological testing is now the comparability of the obtained results with different techniques in different laboratories.

On one hand, laboratories are required to participate in external quality assurance protocols schemes to ensure the comparability of the results. On the other hand, the quantification of autoimmune biomarkers and autoantibodies presents particular challenges because of the nature of the entity measured. Immunoassays rely on detecting the binding of the analyte to its natural antigen. As antigens associated with autoimmune diseases are typically large proteins with multiple epitopes, different immunological testing can detect different epitopes of the same autoantibodies. Consequently, autoantibodies with different epitope specificities will often produce discrepant results depending on the selectivity of the method. Furthermore, the clinical importance regarding an antigen's epitopes is not always known. Where evidence regarding clinically relevant epitopes is available, assay manufacturers should produce appropriate assays.

aPL and their testing

The presence of aPL is currently assessed by solid-phase assays to identify anticardiolipin antibodies and anti-β2GPI antibodies and liquid-phase coagulation assays to identify LA. While a lack of agreement about standard materials and procedures has historically led to a high degree of inter-laboratory and inter-assay variability, in recent years considerable effort has been put into developing international standards for aPL testing.

When considering aPL testing, some considerations are worth noting:

1. LA is a coagulation test: despite significant progress and the updated guidelines of the ISTH (1), LA testing still suffers from some shortcomings and remains much more labour intensive and complicated to perform compared to immunoassays. Is it well-known that one of the major drawbacks of LA tests is their sensitivity to anticoagulant therapy (such as vitamin K antagonists (VKA), and direct oral anticoagulants (DOAC)), due to their interference with coagulation-based assays.

2. aCL and anti-β2GPI antibodies: qualitative agreements between immunoassays for both antibody isotypes are usually acceptable, with almost perfect inter-assay

reliability; however, the correlation between antibody titre and clinical manifestations of APS might be still assay kit-dependent (2, 3).

3. New assays for detecting aPL utilize a variety of approaches; some use traditional ELISA techniques, whereas others use different methods, which could potentially affect their diagnostic accuracy (e.g. chemiluminescence assay, thin-layer chromatography, multiline dot assay). While the level of agreement between ELISA and chemiluminescence assays seems robust, further investigations are needed to explore the clinical accuracy of other techniques for aPL detection.

Risk scoring tools in clinical practice

Risk assessment scoring systems, such as the Global APS Score (GAPSS) (Box 2.5.2), takes into account the combination of independent cardiovascular risk factors and the aPL positivity profile and might help to identify patients with aPL who are at higher risk for developing any clinical manifestations of APS (thrombotic and/or pregnancy morbidity) (4).

Overall, assessment of risk factors for adverse maternal and foetal outcomes in pregnant women with aPL is crucial for preconception counselling and implementing appropriate preventive strategies and a patient-tailored monitoring plan before and during pregnancy.

Pre-pregnancy counselling should be offered to all women with aPL or APS, taking all risk factors into consideration. It may be necessary to recommend postponing pregnancy in order to improve general health and reduce risk, such as the need for weight loss following an acute thrombotic event.

Box 2.5.2 Assessing the risk with the Global APS Score (GAPSS)

The Global APS Score (GAPSS) was created to help assess the risk of developing APS-related clinical manifestations. This score derived from the combination of independent risk factors for thrombosis and pregnancy loss, taking into account the aPL profile (criteria and non-criteria aPL), conventional cardiovascular risk factors, and the autoimmune antibodies profile. It has been demonstrated that risk profile in APS can be successfully assessed, suggesting that GAPSS can be a potential quantitative marker of APS-related clinical manifestations.

Hyperlipidaemia	3
Arterial hypertension	1
aCL IgG/IgM	5
Anti-β2GPI IgG/IgM	4
APS/PT IgG/IgM	3
LA	4

aCL, anticardiolipin; anti-β2GPI, anti-beta2 glycoprotein; aPL, antiphospholipid antibody; APS, antiphospholipid syndrome; LA, lupus anticoagulant.

Box 2.5.3 Suggested points to include in pre-pregnancy counselling sessions in line with current 'EULAR recommendations for women's health and the management of family planning, assisted reproduction, pregnancy, and menopause in patients with systemic lupus erythematosus and/or antiphospholipid syndrome' (1)

- Clinical: review medical and obstetric history
- Laboratory:
  - (a) document and confirm persistent antiphospholipid antibodies
  - (b) assess renal function
  - (c) assess full blood count for presence of thrombocytopenia and/or anaemia
  - (d) antibody testing: aCL, LA, IgG and IgM, anti-β2GPI IgG and IgM, anti-Ro and La antibodies (even if there is no evidence of SLE: these antibodies are associated with a 2% risk of complete heart block in the foetus and up to a 5% risk of neonatal lupus)
- Treatment pre-pregnancy:
  - (a) optimize the woman's clinical state and pharmacological treatment (if any)
  - (b) postpone pregnancy if a thrombotic event has occurred within the last 6 months
  - (c) in case of co-existing SLE, postpone if SLE has been active or hypertensive within the last 6 months
  - (d) assess individual additional risk factors such as obesity, smoking and maternal age and give comprehensive information to the woman regarding the degree of risk for both thrombosis and obstetric complications
  - (e) provide contact information for prompt and early referral at the onset of pregnancy
  - (f) ensure that the management plan is understood, e.g. substituting heparin for warfarin at the time of the first missed period
  - (g) ideally, provide the woman with a supply of LMWH and lessons in self-injection

SLE—systemic lupus erythematosus; LMWH—low-molecular-weight heparin.

A clear plan for pregnancy management should be developed as outlined in Box 2.5.3. Treatment recommendations for women with aPL or APS is outlined in Table 8.3.1 Chapter 8.3.

Case 3: How to counsel a woman with Ro antibodies and a history of a previous pregnancy with congenital heart block (CHB) who is planning a further pregnancy

A 25-year-old teacher is seen in your clinic. She had a baby boy born with congenital heart block (CHB), and she was subsequently found to be positive for Ro antibodies.

She received no treatment during pregnancy, and her baby boy is doing well with a pacemaker. She has no other pregnancy history and no symptoms suggestive of any underlying connective tissue disease. New blood tests confirm her positivity for anti-Ro/SSA antibodies. She would like to plan a further pregnancy. Do you advise any treatment?

Case discussion

CHB is a foetal cardiac injury, detected before, at birth or within the neonatal period caused by transplacental passage of maternal antibodies against SS-A/Ro and SS-B/La (please also see Chapter 1 case 5). The incidence of CHB in the general population varies between 1 in 15,000 to 1 in 22,000 live-born infants. Injury to foetal conduction tissues caused by transplacental exposure to maternal autoantibodies is responsible for 60–90% of cases of congenital CHB overall. Among women with anti-Ro/SSA and/or anti-La/SSB antibodies, foetal/neonatal CHB occurs in approximately 2% of pregnancies. However, once a woman has given birth to an infant with autoimmune CHB block, the recurrence rate in subsequent pregnancies rises to approximately 15%. Foetal surveillance including foetal echocardiography should be offered to these women if possible, but this may depend on local availability. The most vulnerable period for the foetus is during the period from 18–24 weeks' gestation. Normal sinus rhythm (NSR) can progress to complete atrioventricular block within 7 days during this high-risk period. New onset of heart block is less likely during the 26th through to the 30th week, and it rarely develops after 30 weeks of pregnancy. Foetal echocardiography is indicated if there is suspected foetal dysrhythmia or myocarditis, especially in the context of positive maternal anti-Ro/SSA or anti-La/SSB antibodies. Other tests (electrocardiogram plus Holter monitor, magneto-cardiography, gated-pulsed Doppler technique, velocity-based foetal kinetocardiogram) might detect subtle signs of the development of AV block, but are not currently recommended as standard practice. To date, there is no proven efficacy of protocols for the prevention or treatment of complete CHB. The efficacy of maternal fluorinated steroids has not been established in large cohorts despite initial reports of favourable effects in cases of incomplete CHB. A case-control study suggested a benefit of hydroxychloroquine (HCQ) in lowering the risk of cardiac manifestations of neonatal lupus (cardiac-NL), including CHB, in pregnancies of anti-SSA/Ro positive patients with systemic lupus erythematosus (SLE). A historical cohort assembled from three international databases was used to evaluate whether HCQ reduces the nearly 10-fold increase in risk of recurrence of cardiac-NL, independent of maternal health status. Based on these aggregate data from a multinational effort, in mothers at high risk of having a child with cardiac-NL, the use of HCQ seems to protect against recurrence of disease in a subsequent pregnancy and should therefore be suggested.

Anti-Ro/SSA and/or anti-La/SSB antibodies are typically found in patients with SLE or Sjögren's syndrome; however, they can be found also in women with no clinical manifestations of connective tissue disease. While anti-Ro/SSA antibodies are the most prevalent specificity among many autoimmune diseases, serum containing autoantibodies directed against the Ro/SSA antigens may recognize one or both of two cellular proteins with molecular weights of approximately 52 and 60 kD. These autoantigens are referred to as 'Ro52' and 'Ro60', respectively. The two autoantigens were originally thought to interact with each other, but subsequent studies have shown that the two proteins reside in distinct cellular compartments, with Ro60 localized to the nucleus and nucleolus and with Ro52 localized to the cytoplasm. Both autoantigens, Ro52, and Ro60, and La ribonucleoprotein antibodies have been found to increase the risk of giving birth to an infant with isolated CHB (5).

Case 4: How to counsel a woman with U1RNP/mixed connective tissue disease (MCTD) who is planning to become pregnant

A 32-year-old banker is referred to you. She has been told that she is extractable nuclear antigen (ENA) positive but has no other symptoms. She is worried if that has any implications for her wish to have a baby in the future. You take a full history and she explains that she has Raynaud's affecting her fingers mainly in winter. She also has occasional joint aches in her wrists (you suspect that she fulfils Sharp criteria for MCTD). After blood testing, and you confirm her ENA positivity showing a strongly positive U1RNP. She would like to know whether she can have a baby.

Case discussion

MCTD is classified by the presence of high titres of antibodies to U1-RNP in patients with 'puffy hands', Raynaud's phenomenon, arthritis, and myositis. Testing for ENA is mandatory to classify patients with any suspected CTD, particularly when planning a pregnancy.

While there is currently no clear recommendation about pregnancy counselling in women with MCTD and isolated anti-U1RNP, a growing body of evidence suggests that the presence of maternal antibodies to Ro/SSA and/or La/SSB, although a powerful risk factor for CHB and neonatal lupus, is not the only determinant of the development of these complications (6, 7). Maternal antibodies to other antigens may cause neonatal disease in some cases. Anti-U1RNP (small nuclear ribonucleoprotein that associates with U1 spliceosomal RNA) antibodies in the absence of anti-Ro/SSA or anti-La/SSB antibodies were found in a few instances of newborns with neonatal lupus (NL). These patients had the classic rash of NL but no AV block. There are anecdotal reports of heart block associated with anti-RNP but absent anti-Ro/SSA-La/SSB. Recently two interesting observations were two reports of CHB in foetuses born to mothers with MCTD with isolated high-titre anti-U1RNP, who was persistently negative for anti-Ro/SSA and anti-La/SSB (7). When considering the current literature, a recent systematic review (from 1987 to 2018) described 18 cases of NL in patients with anti-U1RNP in the absence of anti-Ro/SSA. Very recently, in a multicentre cohort, women with MCTD had a live birth rate of 72%. While the true frequency of heart block associated with anti-U1RNP remains to be determined and the literature on pregnancy outcomes in women with MCTD is scarce, these new observations might raise the consideration of echocardiographic surveillance and pregnancy counselling. However, more data are needed to support this observation.

Key messages

- A variety of autoantibodies associated with rheumatic diseases have been associated with adverse maternal and foetal pregnancy outcomes.
- aPL-related pregnancy morbidity includes recurrent recurrent 1st trimester pregnancy loss (<10 weeks' gestation) and 2nd or 3rd trimester pregnancy complications including complications related to ischaemic placental dysfunction.
- ENA, such as anti-Ro/SSA and/or anti-La/SSB antibodies, have been associated with the development of CHB and neonatal lupus in the offspring.
- In general women with rheumatological diseases should receive pregnancy counselling and should be tested for the presence of these antibodies prior to pregnancy.

Further reading

1. Andreoli L, Bertsias GK, Agmon-Levin N, et al. EULAR recommendations for women's health and the management of family planning, assisted reproduction, pregnancy and menopause in patients with systemic lupus erythematosus and/or antiphospholipid syndrome. *Ann Rheum Dis.* 2017;76(3):476–85.
2. Lockshin MD, Kim M, Laskin CA, et al. Prediction of adverse pregnancy outcome by the presence of lupus anticoagulant, but not anticardiolipin antibody, in patients with antiphospholipid antibodies. *Arthritis Rheum.* 2012;64(7):2311–18.
3. Saccone G, Berghella V, Maruotti GM, et al. Antiphospholipid antibody profile based obstetric outcomes of primary antiphospholipid syndrome: The PREGNANTS study. *Am J Obstet Gynecol.* 2017;216(5):525 e521–525 e512.
4. Sciascia S, Sanna G, Murru V, Roccatello D, Khamashta MA, Bertolaccini ML. GAPSS: The Global Anti-Phospholipid Syndrome Score. *Rheumatology* (Oxford). 2013;52(8):1397–403.
5. Buyon JP, Hiebert R, Copel J, et al. Autoimmune-associated congenital heart block: Demographics, mortality, morbidity and recurrence rates obtained from a national neonatal lupus registry. *J Am Coll Cardiol.* 1998;31(7):1658–66.
6. Tardif ML, Mahone M. Mixed connective tissue disease in pregnancy: A case series and systematic literature review. *Obstet Med.* 2019;12(1):31–7.
7. Radin M, Schreiber K, Cuadrado MJ, et al. Pregnancy outcomes in mixed connective tissue disease: A multicentre study. *Rheumatology* (Oxford). 2019;58(11):2000–8.

SECTION III
ADJUSTMENT OF THERAPY BEFORE/DURING PREGNANCY AND LACTATION

3.1
Adjustment of therapy before/during pregnancy and lactation

Monika Østensen and Ian Giles

Introduction

Medication usage during pregnancy and lactation is a challenge for patients and doctors alike. Advising pregnant women about the safety of medication use during pregnancy and lactation is complicated by a lack of data necessary to engage the woman in an informed decision. Fear to harm the foetus or the nursing baby by maternal drug treatment has resulted in reluctance to administer medicines to pregnant and lactating women. Often, adequate safety data are lacking. However, limited evidence of safety is not automatically evidence for harm. Health care providers (HCP) need to recognize that not treating active rheumatic disease also carries substantial risks for mother and child. Uncontrolled disease may expose the mother to disease progression and organ damage and impair normal growth and development in the foetus. Patients and their partners should be informed that independent from medication, there is a 3–5% background risk in every pregnancy of having a baby with a birth defect. Information on medication use during pregnancy and lactation should be given in a language understandable for lay people to secure compliance with treatment.

During pregnancy, a balance must be struck between maintenance of adequate drug levels required to control disease activity and a reduction in drug levels towards the lower end of the therapeutic range in women who remain in stable remission. There are obvious risks in electively changing an effective drug immediately prior to or during pregnancy in the absence of an adverse effect. This is because any change in medications may result in increasing disease activity, and data suggest that stable disease is one of the most important predictors regarding pregnancy outcomes. Following any change in immunosuppressives prior to pregnancy, patients should be observed for their response and, ideally, they should remain in remission for at least 6 months prior to conception.

Decisions on medications should be made on a case-by-case basis, as the short- and long-term effects of foetal exposure are often poorly characterized. Drug clearance may also be prolonged in neonates. Therefore, each case must be evaluated carefully to balance the decision of drug use during pregnancy on risks and benefits for the mother and the child.

Breastfeeding: many women with rheumatic diseases do want to breastfeed. However, active disease during pregnancy or fear of a postpartum flare may result in not initiating breastfeeding or to limit duration of breastfeeding. HCP unfamiliar with drug pharmacokinetics during lactation may recommend weaning when medication is restarted after delivery at a disease relapse. Unfortunately, many misconceptions remain regarding drugs during lactation, leading to discontinuation of therapies which are of low risk. Breastfeeding initiation and duration could be optimized by improving the level and quality of information provided to patients and their care givers.

Male patients have become increasingly aware of possible effects of medications on their reproductive health. At present, drug effects on male fertility and child outcome are also poorly characterized. For many agents used to treat rheumatic diseases knowledge of consequences of paternal use on reproduction is sparse or even absent.

The following paragraphs deal with different drug classes: traditional disease-modifying drugs (DMARDs), biological agents, and concomitant medications administered for symptoms or comorbidities in patients with multisystem rheumatic diseases, see Table 3.1.1.

Table 3.1.1 Classical and targeted disease-modifying drugs during pregnancy and lactation

Drug	Use in pregnancy	Comments	Compatible with lactation	Comments
Hydroxychloroquine	**Yes**; keep dose at 5 mg/kg/day		**Yes**	Eye checks should be performed according to local guidelines
Sulfasalazine	**Yes**; keep dose at 2 g/day	Folic acid substitution	**Yes**	Folic acid substitution in mother
Azathioprine	**Yes**; keep dose at 2 mg/kg/day		**Yes**	
Ciclosporin	**Yes**; keep dose at 2.5–3.5 mg/day	Control blood pressure and renal function	**Yes**	
Tacrolimus	**Yes**	Measure trough levels	**Yes**	
Leflunomide	**No**; but no proof of human teratogenicity	Washout before planned pregnancy recommended	**Avoid**—lack of data	
Colchicine	**Yes**; dose 1 mg/day		**Yes**	
Prednisone	**Yes**; keep dose between 2.5–7.5 mg/day if possible	Intraarticular injections and intramuscular injections can be given in pregnancy	**Yes**	When using ≥20 mg/d delay breastfeeding until 4 hr after last dose

Table 3.1.1 Continued

Drug	Use in pregnancy	Comments	Compatible with lactation	Comments
Teratogenic drugs				
Methotrexate	No; increases miscarriage rate and birth defects	Discontinue 1–3 months before pregnancy; continue folic acid substitution	Use during lactation may be considered	Minimal excretion into breastmilk
Mycophenolate mofetil	No; increases miscarriage rate and birth defects	Discontinue 6 weeks before pregnancy	**Avoid**—lack of data	
Cyclophosphamide	No; teratogenic in 1st trimester; use at life-threatening maternal disease in 2nd/3rd trimester possible	Discontinue 3 months before pregnancy	**No**	
Targeted therapies				
Apremilast	**Avoid**—lack of data	Prospective study ongoing	**Avoid**—lack of data	
Tofacitinib	**Avoid**—limited data from safety data base	Preliminary data show no increase of miscarriage or birth defects	**Avoid**—lack of data	
Baricitinib	**Avoid**—lack of data	Contraception during therapy and 1 week after stop recommended	**Avoid**—lack of data	

How to adjust traditional DMARDs/immunosuppressives in pregnancy

Case 1: Rheumatoid arthritis (RA) on peroral methotrexate (MTX) experiences accidental conception and 1st trimester exposure to MTX

A 29-year-old hairdresser has been diagnosed with seronegative rheumatoid arthritis (RA) 19 months ago. She was referred to a rheumatologist and was started on peroral methotrexate (MTX) 20 mg once weekly which has controlled arthritis in the small joints of her hands. Before prescription of MTX both oral and written information on side effects of MTX was given and the necessity of effective birth control was discussed. Supplementation of folate 1 mg/day was initiated. The patient had regular 3-months visits during the first year of RA but has since met more irregularly. She lives with her husband and a daughter of 4 years.

The patient phones her rheumatologist and tells that she has taken a pregnancy test which was positive. Ultrasound examination has confirmed a 7 weeks' pregnancy. Her last dose of 20 mg MTX was at week 6 of gestation. The patient is anxious about possible harmful effects on the baby. At the same time, she expresses the wish to have a second child. She asks whether it is possible to find out whether harm has been done and how she should proceed now.

Case discussion

Low-dose MTX (5–25 mg/week) is the standard of care for RA and other inflammatory arthritides like juvenile idiopathic arthritis, psoriatic arthritis, and spondyloarthritis. In any cases of unintended MTX exposures during early pregnancy, it is important to ascertain the exact time of exposure and the exact time of conception (see Chapter 3.2).

The challenge in this case is whether 20 mg MTX at week 6 is embryotoxic. Exposure during gestational weeks 5–8 has been suggested as critical, however, the exact malformation rate after 1st trimester exposure to MTX is unknown. Likewise, the critical dose (if any) for inducing malformations is not known. The most severe malformation is the foetal MTX syndrome consisting of multiple central nervous system, skeletal, and cardiac abnormalities. From several studies including about 200 pregnancies with low-dose once-weekly exposure the malformation rate was between 5–10%. It appears from a prospective study in patients with RA that MTX use up to 6 weeks preconception does not increase spontaneous miscarriage or congenital malformations. However, when given at doses between 10–20 mg/week during the 1st trimester, a high rate of spontaneous miscarriage (20–43%) and an increase in congenital malformations with a variety of single and combined defects has been observed. Two major consensus papers by the European League against Rheumatism (EULAR) and the British Society for Rheumatology (BSR) have concluded that MTX must be stopped 1 to 3 months before a planned pregnancy.

As mentioned previously, it is critical for the risk assessment in this patient to know the compliance and exact time of the last MTX dose in relation to the first day of the last menstrual period to evaluate whether 1st trimester exposure has actually occurred. Prenatal testing by amniocentesis or chorionic villus sampling can assess for neural tube defects and other chromosomal anomalies. A detailed ultrasound assessing growth, skeletal, and other anomalies should be performed by an experienced expert of foetal medicine at the beginning of the 2nd trimester and around week 18–20 to detect birth defects associated with MTX. Despite that ultrasound is not able to detect all potential problems caused by MTX exposure, the risk for anomalies is small. This should be discussed with the patient to facilitate informed decisions. The preferences and values of the patient should be respected.

> Patients who had good effect of MTX sometimes ask whether they can restart MTX after the 1st trimester or during lactation.

No long-term follow-up of children exposed to MTX in late pregnancy exist, therefore MTX should be avoided even after the 1st trimester. Brain development and growth continue throughout the 2nd and 3rd trimester and growth restriction or learning problems could result from MTX exposure in pregnancy.

Experts do not agree on MTX during breastfeeding. Some argue that weekly low-dose 10–20 mg MTX does no harm to the breastfed infant. Case reports have described the very limited excretion of MTX into breastmilk with exposure to <1% of the maternal weight adjusted dose in the breastfed infant. Given its lipid-insoluble nature, MTX may be considered during lactation.

Case 2: Accidental conception and 1st trimester exposure to leflunomide

A 28-year-old female patient with seropositive RA treated with low-dose prednisone and leflunomide (LEF) for one year informs her rheumatologist that she is 6 weeks pregnant. The patient had two spontaneous 1st trimester miscarriages 2 years ago. After the pregnancy test was positive, her gynaecologist ordered bedrest for a pregnancy at risk. She did not carry out the recommended washout procedure for LEF with cholestyramine. Her physician asks whether she can safely carry on with the pregnancy. The patient refuses to do a washout now because she thinks it can jeopardize the pregnancy and lead to a new miscarriage.

Case discussion

At present it is not known whether LEF increases the risk of birth defects in humans because the overall number of exposed pregnancies remains small (<250). Warnings were issued after the introduction of LEF related to pregnancy studies in animals showing an increased risk of birth defects at pharmacological doses comparable to those used to treat humans. The manufacturer has therefore advised safe birth control while on treatment and a washout with cholestyramine or charcoal of LEF when planning a pregnancy.

The clearance of LEF from the body varies amongst individuals from 2–3 months up to 2 years. Therefore, a washout procedure with cholestyramine or active charcoal to enhance elimination of LEF is recommended, achieving a blood level of <0.02 µg/ml in about 2 weeks. The washout should be done before a planned pregnancy or early in the 1st trimester in the case of accidental exposure.

In this case the patient declined a washout for fear of miscarriage. With the present state of knowledge, we have no evidence for or against a washout. Nearly 2/3 of the reported 1st trimester exposed pregnancies (225 cases) reported in the literature underwent a cholestyramine washout. There was no increase in spontaneous miscarriages or birth defects nor a distinct pattern of birth defects common to infants exposed to LEF in the 1st trimester regardless of having a washout procedure or not.

These studies give some reassurance for pregnancies that unintentionally occur while the mother is taking LEF. Until larger and longer-term studies are done, avoidance of LEF during pregnancy is prudent. This patient should be advised to stop LEF immediately, but termination of pregnancy is not indicated. Initiation of another DMARD is indicated to keep her disease activity under control. In case the patient feels insecure regarding possible harm to her baby by LEF, ultrasound checks of the foetus between week 12–14 and a second one around week 18–20 should be arranged to confirm normal development. The patient may be reassured that published evidence thus far has not revealed an increased risk of congenital anomalies caused by LEF.

Case 3: Systemic lupus erythematosus (SLE) patient on hydroxychloroquine (HCQ), azathioprine (AZA), and prednisone during pregnancy and lactation

A 23-year-old patient had onset of SLE with malar rash, arthritis, oral ulcers, fatigue, and lymphopenia. She responded well to a combination of hydroxychloroquine (HCQ), azathioprine (AZA), and prednisone 7.5 mg/day. Episodes with arthritis have been treated with diclofenac, but she does not take it on a daily basis. At age 25, she married and wanted to have children. At a pre-conception visit the patient asks whether she should stop HCQ and AZA and only continue prednisone, adjusting the dose according to symptom severity. She wants to know whether taking diclofenac at a relapse of arthritis would be possible. She plans to breastfeed and wants to know which of her medications are compatible with lactation.

Case discussion

The patient should continue HCQ, AZA, and prednisone throughout pregnancy. HCQ exerts major benefits and should be given to all women with SLE whether pregnant or not. The dose of 200 mg once or twice daily (up to 5 mg/kg per day) should be kept also in pregnancy. Several cohort studies have clearly shown that maintenance of HCQ before and throughout pregnancy prevents lupus flares, reduces the risk of neonatal lupus syndromes, and even the recurrence of congenital heart block. HCQ has been proposed to prevent the thrombotic effects of anti-phospholipid antibodies. It can counteract some of the adverse effects of chronic corticoid use by lowering serum total cholesterol and serum low-density lipoprotein cholesterol (LDL-C) levels. There is some indication that HCQ lowers the risk of pre-eclampsia, pre-term delivery, and intrauterine growth restriction (IUGR). Follow-up studies of in utero exposed children have not shown visual, hearing, growth, or developmental abnormalities.

Vast experience on the use of AZA and its active metabolite 6-mercaptopurine (6MP) in pregnant women with organ transplants, inflammatory bowel disease (IBD), SLE, and other autoimmune disorders has not shown an increase in congenital malformations. Outcomes like prematurity and intrauterine growth restriction have been observed but ascribed to the underlying maternal pathology and disease severity. AZA can induce lymphopenia and transient immunodeficiency in antenatally exposed children; therefore, the dose of AZA should be kept at 2 mg/kg/day.

Conventional non-steroidal anti-inflammatory drugs (NSAIDs), such as ibuprofen, diclofenac, and naproxen, are generally safe in pregnancy but should be avoided in the last trimester due to the risk of premature closure of the ductus arteriosus and used with caution in the 1st trimester due to possible low risk of miscarriage. COX-2 selective NSAIDs (such as etoricoxib) are not recommended due to lack of data and risks identified from animal rather than human exposure.

Other drugs available to treat musculoskeletal pain in pregnancy are shown in Table 3.1.2. Paracetamol has been regarded the first-choice analgesic for pregnant women and been used for decades without any obvious harmful effects on the baby. Intermittent use, however, is advised because some studies have shown links between paracetamol use in pregnancy and an increased risk of wheeze and childhood asthma, cryptorchidism, as well as problems with learning and behaviour in the child. A causative link, however, between these problems and exposure to paracetamol in pregnancy remains unproven. Codeine is compatible peri-conception and throughout pregnancy for acute pain. Several guidelines state that there is no consistent evidence to recommend a dose reduction pre-delivery but neonatologists should be aware of maternal use. For patients in whom amitriptyline, gabapentin, or pregabalin are being used to treat chronic pain, amitriptyline may be continued in pregnancy but gabapentin or pregabalin are not recommended.

Table 3.1.2 Demonstrating alterations in concomitant medication before/during pregnancy with safe alternatives

Indication	Compatible with pregnancy	Contraindicated	Timing of switch before/during pregnancy
Thromboprophylaxis	Low-dose aspirin Heparin	Warfarin Apixaban Rivaroxaban Dabigatran Fondaparinux	Switch to LMWH at confirmation of pregnancy
Hypertension	Labetolol Methyldopa Nifedipine	ACE inhibitors ARBs Chlorothiazide diuretics	Switch to compatible drug at planning/ confirmation of pregnancy
Analgesia	Paracetamol Conventional NSAIDs (up to 32 weeks pregnancy) Amitriptyline Opiates	COX-2 inhibitors Gabapentin Pregabalin	Switch to compatible drug when pregnancy planning

ACEi, angiotensin converting enzyme inhibitor; ARBS, angiotensin II receptor blockers; COX-2, cyclooxygenase-2; LMWH, low-molecular-weight heparin; NSAIDs, non-steroidal anti-inflammatory drugs.

Breastfeeding: the patient can continue HCQ, AZA, and prednisone during breast-feeding. The small amounts of prednisone secreted into breastmilk seem of no clinical importance for the breastfed infant. With high maternal doses (>40 mg/day of predni-sone) consider breastfeeding timing 3–4 hours after maternal drug administration to decrease the dose received by the infant.

Small amounts of AZA/6-mercaptopurine enter breastmilk. The peak concentra-tion in breastmilk is reached 1–2 hours after the mother's last dose with rapid decline of concentration thereafter. Most babies whose mothers chose to breastfeed while taking AZA have been found to have normal blood counts, and they do not have higher rates of infection.

HCQ has been detected in breastmilk in small amounts, but harmful effects have not been reported in a limited number of infants whose mother breastfed while taking HCQ, see Table 3.1.1.

How to adjust biological agents in pregnancy

Case 1: Selection of a tumour necrosis factor (TNF) inhibitor appropriate for use in a subsequent pregnancy

A 31-year-old woman with a 2-year history of rheumatoid factor, anti-citrullinated peptide antibodies (ACPA) positive RA contacts her rheumatologist for counselling. She plans a pregnancy within 1 year. Because of her wish to start a family, initial treatment after diagnosis was with a combination of sulfasalazine and HCQ, periodically supplemented with a NSAID. The degree of improvement of joint symp-toms was sub-optimal, therefore the NSAID was discontinued and a reducing dose of prednisone from 15 mg/day was added to the combination. However, no perma-nent low disease activity was achieved. Consequently, the rheumatologist considers a change from the DMARD combination to a TNF inhibitor (TNFi) and discusses the types of TNFi available with the patient. The patient wants to know whether a TNFi can be used throughout pregnancy without any harm for the baby.

Case discussion

The task is to select a TNFi appropriate for use in a subsequent pregnancy. At pre-sent, five TNFi infliximab, etanercept, adalimumab, certolizumab pegol (CZP), golimumab, and biosimilars of infliximab, etanercept, and adalimumab are available. They differ in structure, half-life, and administration. Infliximab and biosimilars, adalimumab and biosimilars, and golimumab are complete monoclonal immuno-globulin G (IgG1) antibodies, etanercept and biosimilar is a fusion protein containing the crystallizable fragment (Fc) region of IgG1 and certolizumab is a pegylated Fab fragment without a Fc region. Etanercept has a half-life of 2–4 days and must be ad-ministered once weekly or bi-weekly. The other TNFi have a 10–14 day half-life. No pregnancy data are published for the biosimilars of infliximab, adalimumab, and etanercept.

The use of TNFi in patients planning a pregnancy needs to consider the differences in placental passage of TNFi. When administered in the second half of pregnancy, cord blood levels of complete monoclonal antibodies exceed maternal levels at term. Levels of etanercept are much lower because of low affinity of the Fc region to the foetal Fc receptor which is responsible for the active transport of IgG through the placenta. Placenta passage is negligible for CZP even at treatment throughout pregnancy because it lacks a Fc region. For a patient planning a pregnancy a TNFi with low or minimal placenta passage should be selected.

Studies investigating exposure to TNFi throughout pregnancy or during the 2nd and 3rd trimester found an inverse correlation between the time from last exposure to infliximab and adalimumab during pregnancy and drug concentration in the umbilical cord. Drug clearance was prolonged in the newborns, 1.2 times for adalimumab, and 2 times for infliximab. A similar behaviour must be expected from their biosimilars. Low to minimal concentrations in cord blood have been found for etanercept and certolizumab, with the latter found to be below the detectable level in most exposed children.

Data from a large IBD cohort and several studies in rheumatic diseases support the continuation of TNFi throughout pregnancy in patients with active disease to improve pregnancy outcomes. Withdrawal of a TNFi early in pregnancy and before gestational week 24 may result in a disease flare and the necessity to restart immunosuppressive therapy. However, continuation of TNFi could result in immunosuppression in the neonate. Two large cohort studies of infants exposed to TNFi in the 3rd trimester gave different results: one showed a modest increase of infection at 12 months of age, the other showed no increase in the infection rate during the first year of life. In general, mothers who have received biological drugs in mid- to late pregnancy that may cross the placenta at significant levels should be advised to avoid live vaccines in the exposed infant until they are at least 6 months of age, although routine inactivated immunizations should be given as normal.

Case 2: Adult Still's disease refractory to standard treatment and pregnancy

A 25-year-old woman has suffered from adult onset Still's disease (AOSD) for 5 years. The disease has shown a relapsing course. During the last 2 years high-dose prednisone (0.5 g/kg/day) combined with MTX has not controlled the flares. Attempts to control flares with prednisone in combination with AZA, ciclosporin, or etanercept have failed. Anakinra (an interleukin-1 inhibitor) was initiated at 100 mg/day during a severe flare with pericarditis and pleural effusion and had excellent effect. The patient has continued daily anakinra injections during the last year and has stayed in remission. She meets for a regular control with her rheumatologist and informs him that she is 7 weeks pregnant. Can she continue anakinra during her present pregnancy?

Case discussion

This case highlights the problem which arises when patients are refractory to standard treatment. AOSD is a rare systemic autoinflammatory disease characterized by persistent high spiking fevers, joint pain, and maculopapular rash. Lymphadenopathy, hepatomegaly, and splenomegaly often accompany symptoms. Organ manifestations involve the lungs, heart, or kidneys and may occasionally cause severe life-threatening complications. First-line treatment is corticosteroids, but combination with other immunosuppressive drugs is often necessary as shown in this patient. Medications that block the action of interleukin-1 (IL-1) (anakinra and canakinumab) are often effective in refractory cases.

Data on IL-1 inhibitors in human pregnancy are limited. Studies of anakinra in pregnant animals showed no foetotoxicity even at doses × 100 the therapeutic dose despite detection of anakinra in amniotic fluid. Several case reports and series have described pregnancies in patients with periodic fever syndromes treated with anakinra throughout pregnancy. Four miscarriages occurred. Among the 62 live births, two children had congenital anomalies including renal agenesis. In one case this was related to a mutation also present in the mother; in the second case the birth defect occurred in a mother whose disease was not controlled during pregnancy.

Anakinra is steroid sparing, an important consideration in this patient who previously has been refractory to standard treatment. The EULAR consensus paper states that drugs with limited experience in pregnancy may be considered in cases where no other pregnancy-compatible medication can control the mother's disease activity.

The treating physician should recommend continuation of anakinra in the present pregnancy to keep the patient free of flares and spare her and the foetus from the adverse effects of prolonged high-dose corticoids. The limited but relatively reassuring experience with anakinra in pregnancy should be balanced against the risk of uncontrolled disease and its association with adverse pregnancy outcomes and discussed with the patient to arrive at an informed decision.

Breastfeeding should not be discouraged. The literature reports on 13 infants breastfed by their mothers during therapy with anakinra without any side effects. The mother should also be counselled that if anakinra is continued throughout pregnancy then live vaccines should be avoided in the infant until they are at least 6 months of age.

Case 3: Rituximab (RTX) during lactation

A 32-year-old patient with granulomatosis with polyangiitis had been treated for glomerulonephritis. The patient became pregnant 7 months after the last RTX infusion. She continued 5 mg of prednisone throughout the course of pregnancy which was uncomplicated. She delivered a healthy baby girl at term and breastfed the child. A 1,000 mg infusion of RTX was administered 3 months after delivery because of sinusitis, lung symptoms, and increasing levels of proteinase 3 antineutrophil cytoplasmic antibodies (PR3 ANCA). The patient wanted to continue breastfeeding but wondered whether RTX could influence the vaccination regime for the infant.

Case discussion

When administered after week 16 of pregnancy RTX is actively transported across the placenta by foetal Fc receptors. After the 2nd and 3rd trimester treatment of women with malignant or autoimmune diseases leads to cord serum levels of RTX equal to or 2–3 times higher than maternal levels. There have been reports of infants exposed to rituximab in utero with B cell depletion, neutropenia, lymphopenia, thrombocytopenia, and anaemia at birth. Normalization of B cell numbers in the infants has been described after 2–6 months. Experts agree that live attenuated vaccines should not be given to infants with prenatal exposure to RTX between 6–12 months of age or until serum drug levels in the infant are undetectable. Inactivated vaccines can be given, but measurement of vaccine antibodies may be indicated since RTX does impair vaccine responses in adults (response to pneumococcal and haemophilus vaccination).

Excretion of maternal IgG antibodies into human breastmilk is extremely limited, and maternal IgG levels in milk comprise only about 2% (Table 3.1.3). Intestinal uptake of maternal IgG from breastmilk is not common in humans but may occur at repeated dosing at short intervals. Even when maternal IgG is consumed during breastfeeding, the major part will be degraded by digestive enzymes in the infant's

Table 3.1.3 Biologics in pregnancy and lactation

Biologic	Use in pregnancy	Comment	Breastfeeding
Infliximab	Yes	All have active transport through placenta with high concentrations in cord blood when given in the 3rd trimester	Studies have shown low/ minimal levels of TNF inhibitors in breastmilk: infliximab, adalimumab, golimumab, etanercept and certolizumab are all compatible with breastfeeding
Adalimumab	Yes		
Golimumab	Yes		
Etanercept	Yes	Low placenta passage	
Certolizumab	Yes	Minimal placenta passage	
Biologics with limited pregnancy data			*Biologics with limited or absent lactation data*
Rituximab	Avoid in 2nd/3rd trimester	B cell depletion at 2nd/3rd trimester exposure	1 case report showing minimal amount in breastmilk
Belimumab	Use only in case of severe maternal disease when no other pregnancy-compatible drug can control the mother's disease	Animal studies have not shown increase in adverse offspring outcomes. Human pregnancy experience is limited, but has not shown increase in birth defects at 1st trimester use	Case reports published on RTX, tocilizumab, and ustekinumab. No lactation data on belimumab, secukinumab, anakinra, or canakinumab. General comment: minimal amounts of IgG enter breastmilk—if the child ingests IgG proteins they will probably be destroyed in the GI tract. *Breastfeeding should not be discouraged*
Abatacept			
Tocilizumab			
Ustekinumab			
Secukinumab			
Anakinra			
Canakinumab			

gastrointestinal tract. One case report measured excretion of RTX into breastmilk. Less than about 240 times the amount of RTX present in maternal serum appeared in breastmilk. Unfortunately, corresponding infant's serum levels were not analysed.

In the present case, the mother received her last dose RTX 7 months before conception which means that RTX should have been eliminated from her circulation while being pregnant. The child has not been exposed to RTX prenatally nor during the first 3 months of life. Exposure to RTX through breastmilk is unlikely. Therefore, the child may receive the scheduled vaccination programme including live vaccines.

Case 4: Treatment with certolizumab throughout pregnancy and rotavirus vaccination

A 37-year-old woman with RA has been treated throughout pregnancy with CZP. She has been in remission all the time. She delivers a healthy baby at term. She asks her rheumatologist: 'can I breastfeed my baby? Can my child receive rotavirus vaccination at the age of 6 weeks? Can it follow the usual vaccination schedule?'

Case discussion

CZP has no Fc-region and has therefore no active placental transfer mediated by the foetal Fc-receptor. In a pharmacokinetic study of women ≥30 weeks pregnant receiving CZP, plasma concentrations were measured in 14 mother–child pairs at delivery, and in infants again at weeks 4 and 8 post-delivery. Thirteen neonates had no quantifiable CZP levels at birth (<0.032 µg/mL), and one had a minimal CZP level of 0.042 µg/mL. No infants had quantifiable CZP levels at weeks 4 and 8.

The patient can be allowed to breastfeed. A pharmacokinetic study of 17 lactating mothers receiving CZP (CRADLE: A Multicenter, Postmarketing Study Evaluating the Concentration of Cimzia® in Mature Breast Milk of Lactating Mothers) collected and analysed breastmilk samples after ≥3 CZP doses. Seventy-seven of 137 (56%) breastmilk samples had no measurable CZP. For 4/17 mothers, all samples were below the lower limit of quantification. The relative infant dose calculated was 0.15% of maternal dose; <10% is considered unlikely to be of clinical concern. CZP absorption by infants via breastmilk is unlikely due to its low oral bioavailability and Fc-free molecular structure.

Several studies have examined response to vaccination in children after intrauterine exposure to different TNFi. Serum samples collected from 153 infants included in the Pregnancy in Inflammatory Bowel Disease and Neonatal Outcomes (PIANO) study were analysed for titres of antibodies to *Haemophilus influenzae B* or tetanus toxin; no difference to unexposed children were detected.

Rotavirus causes severe gastroenteritis with fever, vomiting, and diarrhoea. The question is whether the child can receive rotavirus vaccination at 6 weeks of age given the lack of or minimal foetal exposure to CZP. Even if minimal exposure had occurred in utero, CZP would have been eliminated by week 6 from the infant's circulation. The results of the CRADLE study confirm no or minimal appearance of CZP in breastmilk and cannot be regarded as a contraindication for rotavirus vaccination.

One study reported on 40 children exposed to a TNFi (13 exposed to CZP) in the 2nd and 3rd trimester of pregnancy who received rotavirus vaccination. Seven children showed a mild reaction to vaccination; only one child exposed to infliximab had diarrhoea.

The European Union (EU) pregnancy label information of CZP reads:

It is recommended to wait a minimum of 5 months following the mother's last CZP administration during pregnancy before administration of live or live-attenuated vaccines (e.g. BCG vaccine), unless the benefit of the vaccination clearly outweighs the theoretical risk of administration of live or live-attenuated vaccines to the infants.

Based on the data available, the pros and cons of rotavirus vaccination should be discussed with the mother and the decision for or against vaccination respect the mother's preferences.

How to adjust concomitant medications

Case 1: Adjustment of concomitant medications in a patient with systemic lupus erythematosus planning a pregnancy

You are seeing a 32-year-old patient who was diagnosed with systemic lupus erythematosus (SLE) 3 years ago with malar rash, oral ulcers, arthralgia, lupus nephritis plus positive ANA, and antibodies to double stranded (anti-ds)DNA but negative Ro/La and aPL. Her SLE and nephritis have been treated and are now in remission for 12 months on HCQ, AZA at 1.5 mg/kg/day, prednisolone (currently 5 mg/day), and an angiotensin converting enzyme inhibitor (ACEi). She has no other comorbidities and is not taking any other medications. She had one normal pregnancy 5 years ago and would like pregnancy counselling regarding the impact her SLE may have upon a future pregnancy.

You advise her appropriately regarding her SLE and pregnancy (see Chapter 8.1) and reassure her that HCQ, AZA, and prednisolone are safe to continue throughout pregnancy and breastfeeding. Regarding her ACEi you explain that this drug is contraindicated in pregnancy and should be switched to an alternative such as labetalol or nifedipine at first confirmation of pregnancy to maintain her blood pressure at safe levels. Furthermore, she will require monitoring for development of pregnancy induced hypertension, particularly when presenting after 20 weeks' gestation with significant proteinuria (known as pre-eclampsia) with measurement of blood pressure and urine protein at each visit and foetal ultrasound and uterine artery Doppler flow studies as dictated by local obstetric practice.

Subsequently she becomes pregnant, switches to labetalol, and starts low-dose aspirin (LDA) to reduce her increased risk of pre-eclampsia given her SLE, previous nephritis, and concomitant steroid. At 28 weeks of pregnancy, however, she develops a malar rash, arthralgia, worsening proteinuria, and hypertension. Given her rising levels of anti-dsDNA antibodies, falling C3/4 levels, and rash you diagnose a lupus flare and increase her prednisone to 40 mg/day for 2 weeks with a concomitant increase in her AZA to 2 mg/kg/day and add nifedipine to reduce her blood pressure. Her condition improves and laboratory values normalize. Her prednisone is reduced to 20 mg/day over 2 weeks and then to a maintenance dose of 10 mg/day over the next 2 weeks with continuation of her increased AZA dose. Her medication is then maintained for the remainder of pregnancy and she delivers a low-birth-weight baby at 37 weeks of pregnancy.

Case discussion

This case further highlights the management of SLE pregnancy discussed in Chapter 6 and demonstrates the requirement to alter ACEi to a safe alternative. The full drug list of any patient must be reviewed to ensure all medications are compatible with pregnancy. Patients with pre-existing hypertension, who are taking ACEi, angiotensin II receptor blockers (ARBs), and/or chlorothiazide agents must switch these drugs that are associated with congenital anomalies at confirmation of pregnancy to alternative antihypertensive agents, such as labetalol, nifedipine, or methyldopa that are compatible with pregnancy. The addition of LDA is recommended in women with SLE who have an increased risk of pre-eclampsia.

Case 2: Use of direct oral anticoagulants during pregnancy

You are seeing a 29-year-old patient in clinic. She has a history of thrombotic antiphospholipid antibody syndrome (APS) (unprovoked deep vein thrombosis (DVT) and pulmonary embolism 2 years ago) and has been treated with warfarin with an international normalized ratio (INR) maintained between 2 and 3. She dislikes warfarin, however, particularly the regular monitoring requirements. She takes occasional ibuprofen for arthralgia but has no other comorbidities and is not taking any other medications. She has no pregnancy history and would like to discuss switching to a direct oral anticoagulant (DOAC), such as rivaroxaban. Her aPL profile remains persistently positive for lupus anticoagulant by dilute Russell's viper venom time (DRVVT) and Taipan snake venom time (TSVT). She does not have any other autoimmune rheumatic disease and her other autoantibody tests, including ANA, dsDNA, and Ro/La are negative.

Given her thrombotic APS you advise her appropriately regarding her requirement for thromboprophylaxis and monitoring by a multidisciplinary team throughout pregnancy to reduce the risk of further thromboembolic episodes and/or pre-eclampsia in this condition (see Chapter 2.1). You explain that large clinical trials of rivaroxaban in APS have shown conflicting results so it is not currently recommended that patients with APS should be started on this drug. Furthermore, the use of rivaroxaban and other DOAC in pregnancy is not recommended. Therefore, she should remain on warfarin, but because it is also contraindicated in pregnancy she will have to switch to injections of low-molecular-weight heparin (LMWH) as soon as her pregnancy test is positive, and her dose will be increased at around 16 weeks due to an increased plasma volume associated with pregnancy. In addition, she should start LDA before conception and will require uterine artery Doppler scans in her 2nd trimester, given her increased risk of pre-eclampsia (see Chapter 6). You also explain that NSAIDs such as ibuprofen are generally safe but should be used with caution in the 1st trimester due to a possible low risk of miscarriage, and avoided completely after 32 weeks of pregnancy due to adverse effects on the baby. After this counselling she decides to continue warfarin, switches to LMWH on the day of a positive pregnancy test, and is then followed up on a regular basis by an appropriate multidisciplinary team without any complications and delivers a normal weight baby at full term.

Case discussion

This case highlights the requirement to switch existing thromboprophylaxis with warfarin or DOACs to LMWH in pregnancy that is itself a procoagulant state. In patients with pure obstetric APS and thus not receiving anticoagulation outside of pregnancy, dual therapy with LDA and LMWH are commenced in early pregnancy to prevent recurrent aPL-related pregnancy complications. Patients with thrombotic APS (with previous venous thrombosis) however, receiving warfarin outside of pregnancy, must switch this drug to an intermediate or treatment dose of LMWH at confirmation of pregnancy because warfarin is contraindicated in pregnancy due to its teratogenic effects.

There is conflicting evidence of the utility of DOAC in thrombotic APS with equivalence of rivaroxaban being shown with warfarin at suppressing markers of endogenous coagulation generation in patients with SLE and venous thrombotic APS. In contrast, patients with a high-risk triple (anti-cardiolipin, anti-ß2glycoprotein I, and lupus anticoagulant) positive aPL profile and arterial thrombotic APS experienced higher rates of recurrence of thrombosis when treated with rivaroxaban when compared with warfarin. Therefore the European Medicines Agency (EMA) has recently announced that DOAC, including rivaroxaban, should not be initiated in patients with APS and patients already on these drugs for APS should discuss with their doctor whether it is appropriate to continue them based upon consideration of their APS features and the EMA recommendation. In pregnancy, there is insufficient evidence on the safety of the DOACs (such as apixaban, rivaroxaban, and dabigatran) so use of these agents is not recommended and any patient who is already taking them should also be switched to therapeutic LMWH at confirmation of pregnancy.

Case 3: Methotrexate and adalimumab in a man wishing to father a child

During a consultation with a 35-year-old man with a 3-year history of RA who is currently in remission on MTX 20 mg/week and adalimumab, the couple ask you whether it is safe for them to conceive on these medications. He has one 4-year-old child with the same healthy female partner and no known fertility problems. You confirm that they are not taking any other medication and reassure them that both MTX and adalimumab can safely be taken by men trying to conceive without any adverse impact upon their fertility or pregnancy outcomes. He subsequently conceives a child with his partner who then goes on to deliver a full-term healthy infant.

Case discussion

In women, effective disease control with medications that are safe in pregnancy are known to improve pregnancy outcomes. This relationship is less clear in men but fertility and active inflammatory disease may negatively affect sperm quality, hence fertility. It is unknown whether good control of paternal inflammatory disease at conception may also improve pregnancy outcomes. There is limited evidence relating to the impact of DMARDs upon male fertility and peri-conception paternal exposure in men with rheumatic disease. Current guidelines on prescribing antirheumatic drugs in pregnancy from the BSR published in 2016, and more recent systematic reviews (see Further reading), have comprehensively reviewed the existing evidence base in relation to paternal exposure to various antirheumatic drugs. These articles report on use of low-dose (≤20 mg/week) MTX in men and found no impact of MTX on fertility or adverse foetal outcomes in over 1,200 reported paternal exposures compared with non-MTX exposed control pregnancies. These findings all support the BSR guidelines that, based on limited evidence, low-dose MTX may be compatible with paternal exposure. The BSR guideline did not specify a need for men on low-dose methotrexate to use barrier contraception during sexual intercourse with their pregnant partner since the risks of a direct toxic effect on the conceptus by exposure to seminal fluid contaminated by methotrexate have not been quantified and drug levels are likely to be insignificant due to the blood–testis barrier. Similarly, no specific concerns have been identified regarding the safety of paternal exposure to various TNFi including adalimumab and BSR guidelines recommend that infliximab, adalimumab, and etanercept are consistent with paternal exposure.

Case 4: Mycophenolate mofetil exposure and fatherhood

A 29-year-old male patient with a 4-year history of SLE with previous nephritis who is currently in remission on mycophenolate mofetil (MMF) 2 g/day asks you whether it is safe for the couple to conceive on these medications. The patient has a healthy female partner and no known fertility problems. You confirm that they are not taking any other medication and explain that although MMF is not recommended to be taken by women in pregnancy because of a high risk of miscarriage, no problems have been shown from studies of men fathering children whilst taking this drug. Therefore, you recommend that they continue this drug. The couple subsequently conceives a child and the partner then goes on to deliver a full-term healthy infant.

Case discussion

Similarly to case 3, this case also highlights how counselling on family planning should be part of the consultation in men as well as women with rheumatic disease. The BSR guidelines and more recent systematic reviews (see Further reading) have comprehensively reviewed the existing evidence base in relation to paternal exposure to MMF. Reassuringly, evidence from over 200 paternal exposures to MMF does not reveal an increased risk of adverse birth pregnancy outcomes. Therefore, these findings support the BSR guidelines that, based on very limited evidence, MMF is compatible with paternal exposure.

Conclusion

Women with inflammatory rheumatic diseases require specific advice about many different drug therapies while trying to conceive and during pregnancy (see Summary Table in Appendix). During pregnancy, screening, managing active disease and the increased risk of pre-eclampsia are important, particularly in patients with a history of hypertension, RA, or SLE (especially lupus nephritis and APS). It is important to reassure women that with careful planning, monitoring, and treatment, most women with these diseases can have successful pregnancies.

Most antirheumatic drugs appear in small amounts in breastmilk and are of no clinical concern for the breastfed infant. All biologics are large molecules with minimal transfer to breastmilk. Even when ingested they would be destroyed in the gastrointestinal tract of the child. Only cyclophosphamide, leflunomide, and mycophenolate should be avoided during lactation, the latter two because of lack of data.

Men treated with immunosuppressive drugs need counselling on possible gonadotoxic effects. The latter is proven to be dose- and age-dependent for cyclophosphamide. Transient infertility can occur during therapy with sulfasalazine. Other antirheumatic drugs have not shown harmful effects on male reproduction though for several drugs data are scarce.

Key messages

- A switch of drugs with proven harmful effects to the child to pregnancy-compatible medications should be carried out before conception or at recommended time points in pregnancy.
- TNF inhibitors are reasonably safe throughout pregnancy.
- Non-anti-TNF biologics are insufficiently studied but may be considered during pregnancy and lactation at strong maternal indication.
- Administration of biologics during the 2nd or 3rd trimester requires avoidance of live vaccines in exposed infants until 6 months after the last maternal dose.
- Breastfeeding is possible with most antirheumatic drugs except for cyclophosphamide, leflunomide, and mycophenolate mofetil.
- The limited experience regarding gonadotoxic effects of medications in men suggests discontinuation before conception only for cyclophosphamide.
- ACEi, ARB, and chlorothiazide diuretics must be switched to safe alternatives at confirmation of pregnancy.
- LMWH remains the mainstay of anticoagulation in pregnancy.
- TNF inhibitors, MTX, MMF, LEF may all be given to men trying to father a child.
- Lack of data in regard to pregnancy and lactation for a given drug is not proof of harm.

Further reading

1. Flint J, et al. BSR and BHPR guideline on prescribing drugs in pregnancy and breastfeeding-Part I: Standard and biologic disease modifying anti-rheumatic drugs and corticosteroids. *Rheumatology* (Oxford). 2016;55(9):1693–97,doi:10.1093/rheumatology/kev404.
2. Flint J, et al. BSR and BHPR guideline on prescribing drugs in pregnancy and breastfeeding-Part II: Analgesics and other drugs used in rheumatology practice. *Rheumatology* (Oxford). 2016;55(9):1698–1702, doi:10.1093/rheumatology/kev405.
3. Gotestam Skorpen C, et al. The EULAR points to consider for use of antirheumatic drugs before pregnancy, and during pregnancy and lactation. *Ann Rheum Dis.* 2016;75:795–810, doi: 10.1136/annrheumdis-2015-208840.
4. Andreoli L, et al. EULAR recommendations for women's health and the management of family planning, assisted reproduction, pregnancy and menopause in patients with systemic lupus erythematosus and/or antiphospholipid syndrome. *Ann Rheum Dis.* 2017;76:476–85.
5. Mouyis M, Flint JD, Giles IP. Safety of anti-rheumatic drugs in men trying to conceive: A systematic review and analysis of published evidence. *Semin Arthritis Rheum.* 2019;48:911–20, doi: 10.1016/j.semarthrit.2018.07.011.
6. Micu MC, Ostensen M, Villiger PM, Micu R, Ionescu R. Paternal exposure to antirheumatic drugs—what physicians should know: Review of the literature. *Semin Arthritis Rheum.* 2018;48:343–55, doi: 10.1016/j.semarthrit.2018.01.006.

3.2

Managing a patient exposed to a teratogenic drug at different stages of pregnancy

Christof Schaefer

Case 1: Methotrexate (MTX) exposure during an unplanned early pregnancy

A 35-year-old primigravid woman is on 25 mg/week methotrexate (MTX) for the past 3 years. Her RA is stable with this medication. Now, an unplanned pregnancy has been diagnosed at gestational week 7 + 3. She and her rheumatologist are extremely worried about the teratogenic risk of MTX which according to the summary of product characteristics (SmPC) should have been withdrawn at least 3 months before conception. The patient is not willing to accept any risk of adverse pregnancy outcome. Therefore, she intends to terminate pregnancy solely because of concerns of teratogenicity.

Case discussion

According to pertinent risk data, MTX is an evidenced teratogen in humans. However, the distinct pattern of birth defects seen with MTX in cancer treatment and after failed abortive application has not been unequivocally observed after antirheumatic low dose. Nevertheless, observational studies indicate a slightly increased overall risk for birth defects and an increased abortion risk. The patient should be informed that even without MTX exposure, any pregnancy still carries an approximately 3–5% risk of a congenital anomaly. The risk increase caused by her MTX exposure still means that she has a more than 90% chance to deliver a child without major birth defects. A detailed ultrasound around week 12 and again during the 2nd trimester is recommended to confirm normal foetal development. Her treatment should be switched immediately to antirheumatics of choice compatible with a pregnancy such as hydroxychloroquine, sulfasalazine, and glucocorticoids (see Chapter 3.1). If necessary, a tumour necrosis factor (TNF)-alpha blocker with sufficient experience in pregnancy may also be acceptable during the 1st trimester (see Chapter 3.1).

Case 2: May cyclophosphamide be used for systemic lupus erythematosus (SLE) flare during the 2nd trimester of pregnancy?

A 37-year-old pregnant woman taking ciclosporin for SLE develops a severe flare with active nephritis at gestational week 18. Unresponsive to immunosuppressive agents recommended for pregnancy and after a positive experience with cyclophosphamide 5 years before, the rheumatologist asked for the risk of this evidenced teratogen during the 2nd trimester of pregnancy.

Case discussion

It is well established that SLE flares during pregnancy are independent risk factors for numerous adverse pregnancy outcomes including pre-term delivery, pre-eclampsia, and even foetal demise, thus treatment escalation to manage disease activity is warranted. If drugs primarily compatible with pregnancy do not promise effective improvement, cyclophosphamide may be considered as the benefits of rapid treatment of an acute flare are likely to outweigh the risks of 2nd trimester antenatal exposure. By gestation week 18 there is no risk for structural birth defects. Most of the children born after 2nd or 3rd trimester exposure to cyclophosphamide were born healthy. Maternal treatment with cyclophosphamide later in pregnancy has not been associated with an increased risk of foetal malformations, although intrauterine growth restriction may occur and oligohydramnios, premature delivery, and neonatal bone marrow suppression are unusually frequent. Both flare of SLE and maternal cyclophosphamide therapy require close ultrasound monitoring of foetal growth and wellbeing.

True risk vs risk labelling

Although information on drug risks in pregnancy has improved substantially since the thalidomide scandal 60 years ago, individualized risk advice is indispensable for clinical decision making. Often there is uncertainty about how to interpret the available scientific data. For the majority of drugs, experience is still insufficient with respect to their safety in pregnancy. Risk and safety aspects refer to several maternal and infant outcomes such as birth defects, spontaneous abortion, intrauterine growth restriction (IUGR), prematurity, postnatal adaptation, immunosuppression, or impaired neurodevelopment of the child (see Figure 3.2.1). Most pregnancy outcome studies address only a selection of these endpoints.

Formal drug risk classifications or short statements such as 'contraindicated during pregnancy' in package leaflets, SmPCs, or physician's desk reference do not adequately support drug risk perception by health care providers (HCP) and patients. These may lead to an overestimation of risk or simple fatalism, resulting in withholding treatment, poor adherence, or the prescription of insufficiently studied drugs. Overestimation of risk can even lead to recommending termination of pregnancy.

In 2008 the European Medicines Agency (EMA) released a guideline on how to improve drug-risk information in pregnancy in Europe (1). Individual decision making requires quantification and specifications of (birth defect) risks. In cases of absence of developmental toxicity, the amount and quality of data that suggest safety have to be specified. Similarly, the United States Food and Drug Administration has revised its pregnancy labelling mandates (2) to provide more of a narrative about data regarding pregnancy risk with antenatal exposure.

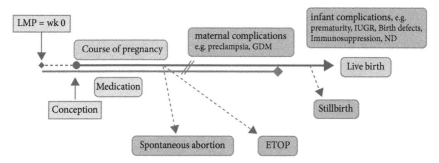

Figure 3.2.1 Course and outcome of pregnancy. This figure gives an overview of the course of pregnancy including the possible outcomes and complications that may be influenced by maternal disease activity and/or medication. ETOP, elective termination of pregnancy; GDM, gestational diabetes mellitus; IUGR, intrauterine growth retardation; LMP, last menstrual period; ND, neurodevelopmental delay.

Prenatal toxicity of drugs in human

Tables 3.2.1 and 3.2.2 give an overview on the most important evidenced teratogens and foetotoxicants in humans with their characteristic clinical features. Table 3.2.3 assigns the disease-modifying antirheumatic drugs to three different categories of evidence of prenatal risk in humans.

Risk communication regarding medication in pregnancy

In general, safety is understood as the absence of risk. Based on this definition, we can hardly categorize any drug as safe because of limited experience. Instead, statements should use the term of relative safety. Information on a drug's risk must support: 1) primary prevention of birth defects and other adverse outcomes; 2) avoidance of overestimation of drug risks resulting in non-prescription or non-adherence; 3) comparative risk assessment between treatment options; 4) comparative risk assessment between medication and untreated disease. Discussion about the risks to the pregnancy that occur due to active systemic inflammation or organ dysfunction due to activity of underlying maternal disease must balance any discussion of risks of medication exposure. Therefore, the trajectory and severity of a woman's underlying disease must be taken into consideration when discussing if and which medications will optimize pregnancy outcomes.

Clinical decision-making should also consider the clinical significance of a hypothesized risk. Recently, the genotoxic potential of hydroxychloroquine was brought up again based on older animal experiments following high-dose parenteral application. Similar findings were also reported for other drugs in the past. The clinical meaning of such experimental findings is difficult to specify. Again, we have to weigh

Table 3.2.1 Most relevant teratogenic drugs with adverse effects after 1st trimester use (e.g. 3, 4, 5)

These drugs do not necessarily harm the exposed embryo. With the exception of thalidomide, retinoids, mycophenolate, and valproic acid, the risk for major birth defects during the 1st trimester does not exceed 10%. Individual risk assessment is recommended in cases of exposure. Substances not listed here must not be regarded as proven safe

Substance	Lead symptoms or predominantly affected organ
Evidenced strong teratogens, with monotherapy risk increase of major birth defects up to 10-fold (30%)	
Retinoids, systemic (acetritin, etretinate, isotretinoin, tretinoin)	ear, CNS, cardiac, skeletal defects
Thalidomide	phocomelia, amelia
Mycophenolate	oral clefts, microtia, aural atresia
Valproic acid	neural tube defects (lumbar spina bifida), radial defects, cardiac, urogenital defects, oral clefts, facial dysmorphia
Evidenced teratogens, with monotherapy risk increase of major birth defects up to 3-fold (10%)	
Androgens	masculinization
Antineoplastic drugs	multiple defects
Carbamazepine	spina bifida, cardiac, urogenital, limb defects, oral clefts, facial dysmorphia
Coumarin derivatives (phenprocoumon, warfarin)	nose, limb defects
Cyclophosphamide	microcephaly, limb defects
Methotrexate*	cranial dysplasia, limb defects, and others
Misoprostol (failed abortive use)	moebius sequence, limb defects
Penicillamine	cutis laxa (rare)
Phenobarbitone/primidone (as antiepileptic)	cardiac, urogenital, limb defects, oral clefts, facial dysmorphia
Phenytoin	cardiac, urogenital, limb defects, oral clefts, facial dysmorphia
Topiramate	oral clefts
Vitamin A (>>25.000 IE retinol/day)	see retinoids
Weak teratogens (risk <<= 1:100 exposed embryos)	
Glucocorticoids (systemic)	oral clefts
Lithium	cardiac defect (Ebstein anomaly, very rare)
Methimazole/thiamazole/carbimazole	choanal atresia, tracheo-esophageal fistula, aplasia cutis
Trimethoprim/Co-trimoxazole	neural tube defects

* low risk with antirheumatic dosage.

Table 3.2.2 Most relevant foetotoxic drugs with adverse effects after 2nd/3rd trimester use (e.g. 3, 4, 5)

These drugs do not necessarily harm the exposed foetus. Individual risk assessment is recommended in cases of exposure. Substances not mentioned in this list must not be regarded as proven safe

Substance	Lead symptoms or predominantly affected organ
ACE inhibitors	oligohydramnios, anuria, joint contractures, skull hypoplasia
Aminoglycosides (parenteral)	oto- and nephrotoxicity
Amiodarone	hypothyroidism
Androgens	masculinization
Angiotensin-I-receptor-blocker	oligohydramnios, anuria, joint contractures, skull hypoplasia
Antineoplastic drugs	IUGR, pancytopenia, developmental delay
Azathioprine	pancytopenia
Benzodiazepines (long-term or during delivery)	apnoea, adaptation disorder, floppy-infant syndrome
Coumarin derivatives (phenprocoumon, warfarin)	cerebral bleeding
Ergotamines (near term or pre-term contractions)	foetal hypoxia
Lithium	floppy-infant syndrome, hypothyroidism
Opioids (long term or during delivery)	withdrawal syndrome
Psychopharmaceuticals	adaptation disorder, serotoninergic symptoms with SSRI
Radioiodine (in therapeutic dosage)	thyroid hypoplasia or -aplasia
Tetracyclines (after 15 gestational weeks)	teeth staining
Thyreostatics	hypothyroidism
Valproic acid	CNS-development impaired/reduced IQ

these hypothetical risks against the risk of other treatment options and the untreated maternal condition. It must also be noted that many published case reports or series that describe congenital malformations following exposure to maternal medication do not necessarily imply causality. Often, when a new medication becomes available, early case reports of adverse pregnancy outcomes receive a great deal of press without necessarily providing the scientific links to actual causality. In most cases, women are exposed to numerous medications at the discovery of an unplanned pregnancy, and the activity of her underlying disease may also play a role in the pregnancy outcomes. When attempting to associate congenital malformations directly to any given medication, teratologists look for a pattern of malformations that suggest a mechanism

Table 3.2.3 Disease-modifying antirheumatic drugs and their evidence of prenatal developmental risk (e.g. 3, 4, 5)

No substantial risk	No evidenced risk in human, but data too scarce or contradictory to recommend as first-line treatment	Evidenced risk
NSAID <28 gestational weeks	Biologics (largest reassuring experience with adalimumab, infliximab, etanercept, certolizumab)	Methotrexate
Prednisone <15 mg/d	Leflunomide (should not be used when pregnancy is planned, washout treatment in cases of unplanned pregnancy)	Mycophenolate
Azathioprine		Cyclophosphamide
Hydroxychloroquine		
Ciclosporin A		
Sulfasalazine		

specific to a given medication (see Tables 3.2.1 and 3.2.2). Nevertheless, early reports may serve as a signal for further investigation before more definitive conclusions about true teratogenicity risks can be estimated.

Counselling drug exposure during pregnancy requires a differential approach depending on the type of inquiry:

1. Recommendation of a drug of choice for a given disease in pregnancy must consider that thousands of pregnant women or their HCP may follow this advice. Even a slight increase in relative risk (RR) for birth defects may be relevant in terms of additional children born with congenital anomalies. As almost half of all pregnancies are unplanned, all women of reproductive age should only be recommended well-established medications. New drugs should be avoided whenever well-established medications are effective and tolerated by the mother and embryo/foetus.

2. In cases of inadvertent exposure during (early) pregnancy a well-grounded individual risk assessment can help to allay unnecessary fears and avoid unjustified invasive diagnostics or termination of pregnancy. If no risk is evidenced or strongly suspected, the woman should be given a straightforward answer: that there is no reason to worry about her pregnancy. Additional prenatal diagnostic procedures, in particular a detailed ultrasound examination, may be recommended.

3. If a baby is born with a birth defect suspected to be caused by a drug, the probability of a causal association should be carefully assessed based on pertinent human study data.

In Table 3.2.4 prednisone and oral clefts are used as an example to demonstrate risk interpretation, depending on the type of inquiry. Calculations are based on a

Table 3.2.4 Communicating a drug's risk from three different clinical perspectives

Clinical situation	Prednisone and oral clefts; prevalence oral clefts 12/10,000; RR of prednisone 1.9
If 10,000 women take prednisone during 1st trimester there will be	11 additional infants with oral clefts
If one pregnant woman has been exposed to prednisone during 1st trimester the risk for oral cleft is	0.23 instead of 0.12%
If a child is born with an oral cleft after exposure to prednisone during 1st trimester the attributable risk is	47%

hypothesized RR of 2.0 for oral clefts after 1st trimester exposure to prednisone (>15 mg/day) and a prevalence (background risk) of oral clefts of 12/10,000.

The importance of the gestational exposure interval

One of the main aspects of a drug's developmental toxicity is the gestational interval of exposure and the dose. Very early drug effects on the pre-implantation stage may cause early embryonic death, extrauterine implantation, or delayed transport of the fertilized zygote. During the so-called 'all or nothing period' until 4 weeks after LMP, surviving pregnancies with birth defects are generally not expected. Either the pluripotent cells repair a toxic insult, or the pregnancy will end. The hypothesized safety of teratogen exposure during this early stage is, however, not applicable for drugs with longer half-life, such as retinoids. A critical phase for the induction of structural malformations usually occurs during the period of organogenesis beginning 4 weeks after the last menstrual period (LMP) and lasting approximately until week 10. Later, during the foetal period a toxicant usually does not cause structural birth defects. However, severe or even lethal functional impairments may occur or disruption of organ development. Some of these anomalies may mimic malformations.

Managing the patient with a flare during pregnancy refractory to pregnancy-compatible drugs

May the evidenced teratogens MTX, MMF, cyclophosphamide, or drugs with inconclusive or insufficient data such as leflunomide or biologics be used in the 2nd or 3rd trimester? A categorical yes or no answer cannot be given. For these drugs a risk in the 2nd or 3rd trimester cannot be definitely ruled out. Weighing the risk of a disease flare not responsive to pregnancy-compatible drugs against the undefined foetotoxic risk of a suspected teratogen or a drug with scarce data, an effective treatment, e.g. with TNF-alpha inhibitors, should not be discontinued uncritically. A decision should be made individually in cooperation with a clinical teratologist considering pertinent toxicity data and the expected individual effectiveness of a treatment.

Conclusion

Safety in terms of 100% absence of risks cannot be concluded for any effective drug, or even in a completely unexposed pregnancy. Therefore, safety should be interpreted as relative among effective treatment options and in comparison to the untreated disease. Drugs with the largest evidence of safety should be preferred during childbearing age since more than 40% of all pregnancies occur unplanned. Clinical decisions require an individual interpretation considering the risk profile of a medication and the gestational interval of treatment. Even in cases of a suspect exposure, the individual risk of developmental toxicity is often low or negligible. Risks of undertreated active maternal disease must balance discussions of medication risks to the pregnancy.

Key messages

- There is no 100% absence of risks for any effective drug in pregnancy.
- Safety should be interpreted as relative among effective treatment options and in comparison to the untreated disease.
- Drugs with the largest evidence of safety during pregnancy should be preferred in women of childbearing age.

Further reading

1. European Medicines Agency. (2008) Guideline on risk assessment of medicinal products on human reproduction and lactation: From data to labelling: https://www.ema.europa.eu/en/risk-assessment-medicinal-products-human-reproduction-lactation-data-labelling.
2. Food and Drug Administration, Department of Health and Human Services. (2014) Content and format of labeling for human prescription drug and biological products; requirements for pregnancy and lactation labeling. *Final Rule*. FDA Federal Register/Vol. 79, No. 233: 72063–103.
3. Schaefer C, Peters P, Miller RKM. (2015) *Drugs During Pregnancy and Lactation*, 3rd ed. New York: Elsevier/Academic Press.
4. Reprotox: https://reprotox.org/.
5. Embryotox database (German): https://www.embryotox.de/.

SECTION IV
INFECTION DURING PREGNANCY

4

Infection in a pregnant patient on immunosuppressive treatment

Maria Rhona G. Bergantin and Sandra V. Navarra

Introduction

Systemic autoimmune diseases must be kept under good control during pregnancy since untreated disease carries its own risks to both the mother and the developing foetus. Whilst infections are an important complication of immunosuppressive drugs used for many autoimmune rheumatic diseases, their clinical manifestations may be masked or absent among immunosuppressed individuals. The relative benefits and risks to the mother and foetus of using particular medications to maintain disease control while effectively treating the infection depends on the specific clinical context and is generally influenced by gestational age and other factors including drug-to-drug interactions. This chapter deals with practical essentials in the management approach to a pregnant rheumatic disease patient on immunosuppressive therapy who develops an infection.

Antirheumatic drugs considered safe in pregnancy and lactation

Rheumatic disease medications which pose minimal foetal or maternal risk include hydroxychloroquine, sulfasalazine, low-dose aspirin, and azathioprine. Selective use of the following medications is allowed during pregnancy: non-steroidal anti-inflammatory drugs (NSAIDs, except during 3rd trimester), glucocorticoids, calcineurin inhibitors like ciclosporin and tacrolimus, intravenous immunoglobulin, and tumour necrosis factor (TNF) inhibitors. Medications which carry moderate to high risk of foetal harm and should be avoided during pregnancy include cyclophosphamide, methotrexate, and mycophenolate mofetil (see Chapter 3.1).

Anti-infective drugs considered safe in pregnancy and lactation

Antibiotic safety depends on the type of antibiotic and timing during pregnancy. Antibiotics generally considered safe during pregnancy include penicillins or amoxicillins, macrolides, and clindamycin. Antibiotics to be avoided during pregnancy include tetracyclines, nitrofurans, sulfonamides, and their derivatives. The use of most antibiotics is considered compatible with breastfeeding. Penicillins, aminopenicillins, clavulanic acid, cephalosporins, macrolides, and metronidazole at dosages at the low end of the recommended dosage range are considered appropriate for use in lactating women. See Table 4.1 for more specific recommendations regarding use of antimicrobial agents during pregnancy and lactation.

Table 4.1 Recommendations for use of antimicrobial agents during pregnancy and lactation

DRUGS	1st trimester	2nd trimester	3rd trimester	Lactation
ANTIBACTERIAL				
Aminoglycoside	R	R	R	R
Cephalosporin				
Cefaclor	A	A	A	A
Cefalexin	A	A	A	A
Cefotaxime	A	A	A	C
Ceftriaxone	A	A	A	C
Cefuroxime	A	A	A	C
Carbapenem				
Doripenem	--------Limited clinical studies----------			
Ertapenem	--------Limited clinical studies----------			
Imipenem	C	C	C	C
Meropenem	C	C	C	C
Glycopeptide				
Dalvabancin	R	R	R	No clinical studies
Oritavancin	R	R	R	No clinical studies
Telavancin	R	R	R	No clinical studies
Vancomycin	A	A	A	C
Lincosamide				
Clindamycin	A	A	A	C
Macrolides				
Azithromycin	C	C	C	C
Clarithromycin	R	C	C	C
Erythromycin	A	A	A	C
Metronidazole	R	C	C	C

Table 4.1 Continued

DRUGS	1st trimester	2nd trimester	3rd trimester	Lactation
Monobactam				
Aztreonam	C	C	C	C
Nitrofurantoin	C	C	R	C
Oxazolidinones				No clinical studies
Linezolid	C	C	C	
Tedizolid	---------Limited clinical studies----------			
Penicillin				
Amoxicillin	A	A	A	A
Benzylpenicillin	A	A	A	A
Co-amoxiclav	A	A	A	C
Flucloxacillin	A	A	A	A
Phenoxymethylpenicillin	A	A	A	A
Piperacillin-tazobactam	A	A	A	A
Polymyxins	-------------Limited or no data available---------			
Quinolones	R	R	R	C
Tetracyclines	R	R	R	C
Trimethoprim-sulfamethoxazole	R	C	R	C
ANTI-MYCOBACTERIAL				
Ethambutol	C	C	C	C
Isoniazid	C	C	C	C
Pyrazinamide	C	C	C	C
Rifampicin	C	C	C	C
ANTIMALARIAL				
Artemether-lumefantrine	R	A	A	No clinical studies
Chloroquine	A	A	A	A
Mefloquine	A	A	A	A
Quinine	A	A	A	C
ANTIVIRAL				
Acyclovir	C	C	C	C
Famciclovir	C	C	C	No clinical studies
Foscarnet	C	C	C	No clinical studies
Ganciclovir	R	R	R	R

(continued)

Table 4.1 Continued

DRUGS	1st trimester	2nd trimester	3rd trimester	Lactation
Oseltamivir	C	C	C	C
Ribavirin	R	R	R	R
Valacyclovir	C	C	C	C
Valganciclovir	R	R	R	R
ANTI-FUNGAL				
Amphotericin B	C	C	C	C
Echinocandins	--------------Limited clinical studies--------------			
Fluconazole	R	R	R	C
Flucytosine	R	C	C	C

A—Allow C—Caution R—Refrain or not allowed

Clinically significant drug-to-drug interactions of anti-infectives with immunosuppressive agents

Potential drug-to-drug interactions are important in a pregnant patient on immunosuppressive treatment who develops an infection requiring an antimicrobial agent. Drug-to-drug interactions may occur through pharmacokinetic (PK) mechanisms leading to altered drug concentrations of either the anti-infective or immunosuppressive drug, or by pharmacodynamic (PD) interactions increasing or decreasing the efficacy or toxicity of the medications. Many significant PK interactions occur through inhibition or induction of the cytochrome (CYP) 3A4 system by anti-infective agents leading to increased or decreased immunosuppressive agent levels, respectively. For example, drugs that inhibit CYP 3A4/5 such as macrolides and azole antifungals will induce a much greater increase in concentration in calcineurin inhibitors like tacrolimus which are reliant on this enzyme for its metabolism. On the other hand, the well-known CYP 3A4/5 inducer rifampicin will potentially decrease the concentration of many drugs including glucocorticoids. Polypharmacy further poses an increased risk especially when adverse effects are additive, e.g. nephrotoxicity, of particular concern among patients with systemic autoimmune diseases like systemic lupus erythematosus (SLE). Software packages like MIMS* and UpToDate* provide useful practical drug interaction checkers.

Case consults

The following selected case consults deal with infections frequently encountered among patients on immunosuppressive medications and are of special concern in pregnancy because of potential to affect materno-foetal outcomes.

Viral infections

Varicella-zoster infections are frequent among patients on immunosuppressive drugs. Viral hepatitis can significantly impact materno-foetal outcomes.

Case 1

A 25-year-old patient with a history of SLE nephritis (class IV) diagnosed 6 years ago. The patient is now stable on maintenance therapy with azathioprine <2 mg/kg, hydroxychloroquine, and prednisolone 10 mg/day. She has a normal renal function and no hypertension. She is well at present and no symptoms to suggest activity of her SLE. She has no previous pregnancy history and is currently 8 weeks pregnant when she sees you in clinic. She has now developed a rash suggestive of chickenpox.

Case discussion

Varicella-zoster virus (VZV), or human herpes virus 3 can affect 90% of non-immune individuals, with an incubation period of 10–21 days. Infections with VZV are frequently seen among individuals on immunosuppressive agents as the virus stays latent in the dorsal root ganglia and can be re-activated, presenting as dermatomal or disseminated infections with or without fever. The virus is considered to be most infectious 2 days prior to the appearance of the maculopapular to vesicular rashes until after the rashes have crusted over and dried. Transmission is primarily via the airborne mode but the virus can also be shed in clothing or beddings. In immune-naïve individuals, primary varicella infection may develop after exposure to individuals with shingles.

Although the US Federal Drug Administration (FDA) included acyclovir, famciclovir, and valacyclovir in the category B drug list (animal studies failed to demonstrate foetal risk, no adequate and well-controlled studies in pregnant women), there are limited data regarding their safety during the 1st trimester of pregnancy. Of these medications, acyclovir is more widely prescribed. It is to be used with caution, especially in early pregnancy, strongly considering the risks and benefits. Beyond 20 weeks of gestation, however, oral acyclovir is recommended within 24 hours of appearance of rashes to reduce the symptomatology and fever associated with the infection. Should the pregnant patient develop severe varicella, i.e. presence of respiratory symptoms, densely cropping vesicles, haemorrhagic rash, bleeding, neurological manifestations, hepatitis, persistent fever with new vesicles >6 days after onset, intravenous acyclovir is recommended regardless of gestational age.

Neither azathioprine nor tacrolimus has known interaction with acyclovir, valacyclovir, and famciclovir.

Aside from standard precautions, airborne and contact precaution should be employed when dealing with VZV-infected patients. In patients with rashes, varicella-zoster immunoglobulin (VZIg) has no proven benefit. For the immune-naïve pregnant with significant exposure to varicella, i.e. staying in the same room for more than 15 minutes or face-to-face contact with infected individuals during the infectious period, VZIg is recommended immediately or within 10 days upon exposure to the index case. In cases of continuous exposure, VZIg is recommended within 10 days of the appearance of rashes in the index cases.

Case 2

During the 1st trimester of an unplanned pregnancy, a 19-year-old with idiopathic thrombocytopenic purpura (ITP) on prednisone 30 mg/day develops active hepatitis C infection. Hepatitis A and B serology are all negative. Previous attempts to reduce her prednisolone dose have resulted in a reduction of platelet counts, thus the patient is maintained on 30 mg/day prednisolone.

Case discussion

In acute infections with hepatitis C, patients are often asymptomatic. Among symptomatic patients however, right upper-quadrant pain, nausea, tea-coloured urine, jaundice, fever, fatigue, anorexia, pruritus, and confusion may be observed. These symptoms often develop within 2–26 weeks (mean 7–8 weeks) after exposure. Transaminitis and bilirubinaemia are present in most cases and the presence of hepatitis C virus ribonucleic acid (HCV RNA) confirms the diagnosis, most especially in those with undetectable antibodies, as the serum levels often become detectable only after 12 weeks post exposure to hepatitis C virus (HCV). The transaminase and HCV RNA levels may fluctuate during acute infection.

Treatment using direct-acting antivirals during pregnancy is not recommended due to lack of safety and efficacy data. Furthermore, spontaneous viral clearance in 10% of postpartum patients may occur, more commonly in symptomatic than asymptomatic individuals. Therefore, in the previous case, no active antiviral treatment is being given.

The risk of maternal to child transmission during pregnancy and breastfeeding is comparable with the general population, hence, breastfeeding is not contraindicated. However, lactating mothers with cracked nipples should take extra precaution due to the possibility of HCV transmission with blood exposure.

Drugs given for chronic hepatitis C infection including peginterferon, ribavirin, glecaprevir/pibrentasvir, elbasvir/grazoprevir, ledipasvir/sofosbuvir, simeprevir, daclatasvir, or sofosbuvir have no known interaction with prednisone. On the other hand, ombitasvir-paritaprevir-ritonavir and dasabuvir potentiate the action of prednisone. Important: none of these drugs are considered safe in pregnancy. Due to lack of data regarding safety and efficacy, direct-acting antivirals are not recommended to be used during pregnancy and lactation.

As the virus is blood-borne, standard precautions should be employed.

One important hepatitis virus which presents as acute hepatic failure more commonly seen in the 3rd trimester of pregnancy is hepatitis E. It may be food- or waterborne or via blood as well as perinatal transmission. The infection is often self-limiting but may present with cholestatic hepatitis (jaundice >3 months) or chronic hepatitis B. As ribavirin is contraindicated in pregnancy, treatment is mainly supportive with the recommendation of reducing the immunosuppressive dosage, if withdrawal is not possible. In those who develop acute hepatic failure, liver transplantation may be required. To reduce the risk of acquiring hepatitis E virus (HEV), travellers to endemic areas should avoid consumption of street food, raw or undercooked food, and unpurified water.

Bacterial and mycobacterial infections

Pneumonias, either typical or atypical, are an important cause of morbidity and mortality among patients on immunosuppressive drugs. Pulmonary and extra-pulmonary tuberculosis (TB) is a growing concern in SLE, particularly in endemic countries.

Case 3

A 26-year-old patient with rheumatoid arthritis (RA) and interstitial lung disease (ILD) is maintained on prednisone 15 mg/day and azathioprine 100 mg/day. Her latest lung function tests have been stable with no significant reduction in her vital capacity; it was therefore agreed in a multidisciplinary team to keep her on the current immunosuppressive doses. She develops *Legionella* pneumonia whilst in the 18th week of her second pregnancy. She recovers after completing 3 weeks of appropriate antimicrobial treatment.

Case discussion

The aetiology of pneumoniae in immunocompromised patients broadens to range from common 'typical' pathogens like *Streptococcus pneumoniae* to unusual pathogens like *Pneumocystis jirovecii*. There is paucity of data regarding the exact incidence of *Legionella* infection in pregnant patients, though in the general population it is considered a significant cause of atypical pneumonia. It often presents with cough, fever, and dyspnea, but there should be a high index of suspicion for the pathogen when the following manifestations are present: diarrhoea, nausea, vomiting, hyponatraemia, elevated C-reactive proteins, transaminitis, and non-response to beta-lactam therapy. Transmission occurs via inhalation of aerosols or aspiration of water laden with the pathogen, often in a common source setting. Incubation period ranges from 2–10 days with median of 6–7 days. To confirm the diagnosis, *Legionella* polymerase chain reaction, urinary antigen, and sputum culture using selective medium may be performed.

The main medications recommended for *Legionella* infections include macrolides, quinolones, or tetracyclines. Amongst these, azithromycin or levofloxacin are preferred due to their bactericidal nature along with high intracellular concentrations and extensive lung tissue uptake. However, only macrolides are considered safe during pregnancy. Quinolone-associated foetotoxicity includes cartilage damage, renal and cardiac toxicity, and central nervous system damage; however recent evidence refutes this, thus, with the conflicting recommendations, it is best to avoid use until further data on safety becomes available.

There are no known interactions between azithromycin and azathioprine or prednisone.

In dealing with patients with *Legionella* infection, observance of standard precaution is recommended. Due to the known mode of transmission, common-source investigation should also be carried out to identify other possible patients.

Case 4

A 28-year-old woman who had undergone a kidney transplant for SLE nephritis progressing to end stage renal disease (ESRD) develops fever in the 2nd trimester of pregnancy. She is diagnosed with pulmonary and genitourinary TB and started on isoniazid, rifampicin, pyrazinamide, and ethambutol. Maintenance medications post-transplant include prednisone 10 mg/day and tacrolimus.

Case discussion

The World Health Organization reports that the burden of TB in pregnancy is substantial with higher incidence in developing countries. If containment of *Mycobacterium tuberculosis* does not occur after inhalation of the droplet nuclei, the host may develop either inactive (latent) or active TB. The clinical manifestations of pulmonary TB in pregnancy are similar to those in non-pregnant patients and may include cough, fever, night sweats, malaise, and weight loss, though the latter may be masked by the expected weight gain in pregnancy due to the developing foetus. Persistent culture-negative pyuria should raise the suspicion of genitourinary TB. Diagnosis can be confirmed by the isolation of *Mycobacterium tuberculosis* via culture of the site-specific specimen, or nucleic acid amplification test (MTb GeneXpert), with the former having the advantage of providing the susceptibility pattern of the mycobacterial isolates which is increasingly becoming important in the face of rising patterns of drug-resistant TB worldwide. Interferon-gamma release assay (IGRA) and tuberculin skin test, on the other hand, may help establish the presence of latent TB infection; however, lower sensitivity may be observed for both tests in pregnancy due to changes in the thymus (T) cell response during pregnancy.

In most countries, pulmonary and genitourinary TB are managed with isoniazid, rifampicin, pyrazinamide, and ethambutol for 2 months (intensive phase) followed by 4 months of isoniazid and rifampicin (continuation phase). If the extrapulmonary site involves bones, joints, or the central nervous system, a total duration of 12 months including a 10-month continuation phase is recommended. Prolongation of treatment duration may also be necessary if the clinical response is slow. Pyridoxine is administered to prevent the peripheral neuropathy often associated with isoniazid.

Rifampicin is a potent inducer of the microsomal enzymes (P450-3A4) that metabolize calcineurin inhibitors, and doses of tacrolimus need to be increased 2- to 5-fold while on anti-TB therapy. Dosing can be based upon trough serum drug levels. Likewise, rifampicin interferes with corticosteroid metabolism requiring an increase of prednisone doses. Rifabutin is a less potent inducer of CYP P450-3A4 and may be used as an alternative to rifampicin. Serum levels of isoniazid may be decreased by prednisone, but similar to pyrazinamide and ethambutol, there are no known interaction with tacrolimus. Pyrazinamide and ethambutol also do not have any significant drug interaction with prednisone.

Precautions against airborne transmission must be observed when caring for patients with pulmonary TB. Bacille–Calmette Guérin (BCG) has no role in TB prevention among pregnant and immunosuppressed patients as it is a live attenuated vaccine.

For patients who have received at least 2 weeks of first-line anti-TB medications, breastfeeding should be encouraged. However, those on rifabutin or fluoroquinolones are advised against breastfeeding.

Fungal infections

Candidiasis is common among immunosuppressed hosts, and vulvo-vaginal candidiasis is especially common during pregnancy.

Case 5

A 30-year-old pregnant patient on prednisone 30 mg/day and azathioprine 150 mg/day for an antineutrophil cytoplasmic antibodies (ANCA) positive systemic vasculitis is seen in your clinic due to oral thrush and symptomatic vulvovaginal candidiasis.

Case discussion

Thrush often develops in individuals with prior antimicrobial treatment, chemotherapy, and those with cell-mediated immune deficiency and on steroids (systemic or inhalational). Vulvovaginal candidiasis is often seen in pregnancy, diabetes mellitus, and in individuals with similar risks for the development of thrush. Patients with oropharyngeal *Candida* may complain of fuzzy sensation inside the mouth, a bland taste or odynophagia, with presence of whitish plaques. Those with vulvovaginal *Candida* infection usually present with vaginal discharge and/or pruritus. Potassium hydroxide preparation (KOH) staining of the plaques or vaginal secretions reveal the presence of budding yeasts with or without pseudohyphae.

A systemic triazole, e.g. fluconazole, is given for 7–14 days in the general population. However, this agent is teratogenic, embryotoxic, and foetotoxic, and thus not recommended anytime during pregnancy. An exception is a single low dose (<300 mg) of fluconazole which may be given after the 1st trimester. Amongst the antifungals, amphotericin B is considered to be the safest during pregnancy, with the nephrotoxicity level similar to that in non-pregnant patients. In cases of superficial mucocutaneous candidal infection, topical azoles may be used as absorption is minimal. Nystatin, however, is best avoided until 14 weeks of gestation.

Fluconazole may increase the serum level of prednisone but there are no reports of interaction between fluconazole and azathioprine. Prednisone may heighten the hypokalaemia in amphotericin B use, hence, serum electrolyte levels need to be monitored. There is no reported interaction between amphotericin B and azathioprine.

Maintenance of oral and perineal hygiene is imperative to prevent the onset and recurrences of oropharyngeal and vulvovaginal candidiasis.

Other infections: malaria, food and water-borne illnesses, leptospirosis

Case 6

A 30-year-old reporter was diagnosed with lupus nephritis (class IV) 5 years prior to her presentation at your clinic. She has been stable on maintenance therapy including prednisone 15 mg/day and azathioprine 100 mg/day. Her blood pressure and kidney function are normal. She is due to travel to parts of Southeast Asia on an assignment and now seeks advice about malaria prophylaxis.

Case discussion

Arthropod-borne

Pregnancy increases the risk for malaria and is attributed to the pregnancy-related immunological and hormonal modifications. Amongst the five species of *Plasmodium*, *P. falciparum* and *P. knowlesi* are associated with severe outcomes in pregnancy though the latter is quite uncommon. *P. vivax*, *P. ovale*, and *P. malariae* are less commonly associated with severe maternal infections. Clinical manifestations are often variable and nonspecific, but fever, chills, headache, excessive sweating, malaise, myalgias, abdominal pain, vomiting, diarrhoea, jaundice, anaemia, and cough are often present. There should be a high index of suspicion, most especially in febrile travellers who have visited a malaria-endemic area. Incubation period varies among species: 12–14 days for *P. falciparum*, 18 days for *P. malariae*, 14 days for *P. vivax* and *P. ovale*. Though some patients may exhibit only mild symptoms, complications such as hypoglycaemia, acidosis, pulmonary haemorrhage, disseminated intravascular coagulation, renal failure, hepatic failure, and coma may be seen in some patients. Microscopic examination of blood smears, malaria rapid diagnostic tests, and polymerase chain reactions are utilized to document the presence of *Plasmodium* spp.

Travel to a malaria-endemic area during pregnancy is best avoided until after delivery. However, if travel is necessary, prophylactic medications are warranted with the use of chloroquine in areas with chloroquine-sensitive malaria, or mefloquine in areas with chloroquine-resistant malaria. Both options are compatible with pregnancy.

Treatment for uncomplicated malaria due to *P. malariae*, *P. vivax*, *P. ovale*, or chloroquine-sensitive *P. falciparum* infection entails the use of chloroquine and hydroxychloroquine at any time. For uncomplicated chloroquine-resistant *P. falciparum* infection, mefloquine *or* quinine plus clindamycin may be given anytime, whereas patients with uncomplicated chloroquine-resistant *P. vivax* malaria may receive mefloquine anytime during pregnancy. Artemether-lumefantrine may be given after the 1st trimester for any *Plasmodium* infection. Tetracyclines are contraindicated at any time during pregnancy.

There are no reported interactions between azathioprine or prednisone with any of the following antimalarial agents: chloroquine, mefloquine, hydroxychloroquine, clindamycin, quinine, and artemether-lumefantrine.

As *Anopheles* species have nocturnal feeding habits, use of mosquito nets (preferably with permethrin) are recommended along with the use of protective clothing (long-sleeved shirts and long pants). Avoidance of mosquito bites is essential.

Foodborne and waterborne diseases

Gastroenteritis with or without pyrexia due to *E. coli*, *Vibrio*, or *Salmonella* may develop secondary to consumption of contaminated food and water. The onset of illness will depend on the burden of microorganisms, the incubation period, and the host's immunity. Confirmation of pathogen relies on stool cultures or polymerase chain reaction when the latter is available. Rehydration is the mainstay of therapy for gastroenteritis to prevent dehydration. If antimicrobials will be needed, macrolides, preferably azithromycin, are the preferred drug as quinolones and tetracyclines are contraindicated in pregnancy.

Azithromycin does not have any known interaction with prednisone or azathioprine.

To reduce the risk of gastroenteritis, travellers are advised to eat only hot and safely cooked food and avoid raw or undercooked food, unpasteurized milk, or fruit juice, unpeeled fruits, and food and beverages obtained from street vendors. Hand washing using soap and water or alcohol-based hand sanitizer is encouraged, most especially during food preparation and before and after meals as well as after using the toilet. Only unopened, factory-sealed bottled water, and boiled and steaming hot beverages should be ingested: avoiding tap water, fountain drinks, and iced drinks.

Leptospirosis

Infection due to *Leptospira* spp. is acquired through exposure of mucous membranes and abraded, non-intact skin to animal urine and contaminated soil and water, often during rainy season when flooding occurs. Incubation period lasts between 2–26 days. Manifestations are variable but often presents with fever, myalgia, calf-tenderness, conjunctival suffusion, and in severe conditions Weil's disease manifesting as bleeding, jaundice, and renal failure. During the initial leptospiraemic phase, bacteria can be isolated from blood and cerebrospinal fluid (CSF); this is followed by the leptospiruric or immune phase, during which antibodies are detectable and organisms may be isolated from the urine. The two phases often overlap and may be indistinguishable. Microscopic agglutination test and enzyme-linked immunosorbent assay (IgM ELISA) for leptospirosis may support the clinical diagnosis.

For mild leptospirosis, the pregnant patient may be given either amoxicillin, ampicillin, or azithromycin. For moderate to severe cases, intravenous medications such as penicillin, ceftriaxone, or cefotaxime are warranted. Treatment is given for 7 days. Doxycycline is contraindicated in pregnancy.

Neither azathioprine nor prednisone has known interaction with any of these medications: amoxicillin, ampicillin, azithromycin, ceftriaxone, cefotaxime, or penicillin.

To prevent leptospirosis, avoidance of animal urine and contaminated soil and water are necessary. Use of rubber boots during the rainy season in flood-prone areas should be observed. For short-term exposure, once weekly azithromycin may be used by the pregnant patient as prophylaxis. Leptospirosis vaccines for humans are only available in select countries, though animal vaccination is widely available.

Key messages

- Both autoimmune disease and infection should be adequately controlled to achieve optimal pregnancy outcomes.

- Clinical manifestations of an infectious disease may present atypically or be obscured among immunosuppressed hosts.
- Certain immunosuppressive and anti-infective drugs have established safety during pregnancy and lactation. There is insufficient data for some medications, particularly novel agents.
- Potential interactions between immunosuppressives and anti-infectives are important to consider in pregnancy.
- Detailed drug monographs and software prescribing packages are readily available to guide decisions in individual clinical situations. Whenever possible, older medications with established safety in pregnancy and lactation should be used preferentially.
- Benefit-risk assessment should be thoroughly discussed with the patient by the attending team of clinicians in coordination with nursing and pharmacy personnel.

Further reading

1. AASLD-IDSA Guidance Panel. Hepatitis C Guidance 2018 Update: AASLD-IDSA recommendations for testing, managing, and treating Hepatitis C virus infection. *Clin Infect Dis.* 2018;67:1477–92.
2. Arguin P, Tan KR. Malaria, [website] 2018. https://wwwnc.cdc.gov/travel/yellowbook/2018/infectious-diseases-related-to-travel/malaria#1939, [accessed 18 May 2019].
3. Kar P, Mishra S. Management of hepatitis B during pregnancy. *Expert Opin Pharmacother.* 2016;17(3):301–10. doi: 10.1517/14656566.2016.1118051.
4. Lateef A, Petri M. Systemic lupus erythematosus and pregnancy. *Rheum Dis Clin North Am.* 2017;43(2):215–26. doi: 10.1016/j.rdc.2016.12.009.
5. Morof DF, Dale Carroll I. Pregnant Travelers [website] 2018. https://wwwnc.cdc.gov/travel/yellowbook/2018/advising-travelers-with-specific-needs/pregnant-travelers, [accessed 18 May 2019].
6. Phin N et.al. Epidemiology and clinical management of Legionnaires' disease. *Lancet Infect Dis.* 2014;14:1011–21.
7. Pilmis B, Jullien V, Sobel J, et al. Antifungal drugs during pregnancy: An updated review. *J Antimicrob Chemother.* 2015;70:14–22.
8. Puchner A et al. Immunosuppressives and biologics during pregnancy and lactation: A consensus report issued by the Austrian Societies of Gastroenterology and Hepatology and Rheumatology and Rehabilitation. *Wien Klin Wochenschr.* 2019;131(1–2):29–44. doi: 10.1007/s00508-019-1448-y. Epub 2019 Jan 14.
9. Royal College of Physicians of Ireland, National Clinical Programme for Obstetrics and Gynaecology. Medication guidelines for obstetrics and gynaecology. *Antimicrobial Safety In Pregnancy and Lactation.* 2017;2. https://rcpi-live-cdn.s3.amazonaws.com/wp-content/uploads/2018/06/Medication-Guidelines_Vol-2_Antimicrobial-safety-in-Pregnancy-and-lactat.._.pdf [accessed 22 May 2019].
10. Royal College of Obstetricians and Gynaecologists. *Chickenpox in Pregnancy Green-top Guideline No. 13.* National Institute for Health and Care Excellence, United Kingdom, 2015.
11. Sparkes T, Lemonovich TL, AST Infectious Diseases Community of Practice. Interactions between anti-infective agents and immunosuppressants—Guidelines from the American

Society of Transplantation Infectious Diseases Community of Practice. *Clin Transplant.* 2019;33(9):e13510. doi: 10.1111/ctr.13510. [Epub ahead of print accessed 22 May 2019].

12. Subramanian K, Theodoropoulos NM. *Mycobacterium tuberculosis* infections in solid organ transplantation: Guidelines from the Infectious Diseases Community of Practice of the American Society of Transplantation. *Clin Transplant.* 2019;33(9):e13513. doi: 10.1111/ctr.13513 [accessed 22 May 2019].

13. World Health Organization (WHO). Malaria in Pregnancy. *WHO Evidence Review Group Meeting Report. Malaria Policy Advisory Committee Meeting.* 2015:1–37. https://www.who.int/malaria/mpac/mpac-sept2015-erg-mip-report.pdf?ua=1ext.

14. Pilmis B, et al. Antifungal drugs during pregnancy: An updated review. *J Antimicrob Chemother.* 2015;70(1):14–22.

SECTION V
ORGAN-SPECIFIC FLARES DURING PREGNANCY

5

Managing organ-specific flares

Bonnie L. Bermas and Eliza Chakravarty

Introduction

Caring for women with rheumatic diseases during pregnancy is challenging. Disease can flare, can be stable, or can go into remission, moreover it is often impossible to predict how a particular patient's disease will fare. At baseline, patients have disparate organ involvement, further complicating clinicians' ability to predict disease course during pregnancy. For example, one patient with systemic lupus erythematosus (SLE) may have mild skin and arthritis manifestations and be at low risk for disease flare during pregnancy, while another patient may have a history of recently active kidney disease, putting her at high risk for flare and pregnancy complications. Furthermore, different organ manifestations can have different impacts on pregnancy. While a flare of inflammatory arthritis during pregnancy can be difficult to manage from a symptom perspective, and may increase the risk of pre-eclampsia and pre-term delivery, it does not lead to the same degree of morbidity or mortality as a lupus nephritis flare during pregnancy might.

Rheumatic disease management during pregnancy is further complicated by the fact that common symptoms of pregnancy such as fatigue, joint pain, and oedema can mimic rheumatic disease flare (Box 5.1). Moreover, laboratory tests that we often use to evaluate and monitor disease activity, such as levels of erythrocyte sedimentation rate (ESR), C-reactive protein (CRP), and complement components, can increase during pregnancy and thus are less reliable indicators of disease flare. Pregnancy itself induces a physiological anaemia, this too can confuse interpretation of laboratory data. Finally, pre-eclampsia, a well-recognized pregnancy complication that occurs at higher frequency in women with rheumatic diseases, can be difficult to distinguish from SLE flare (Table 5.1).

The basic tenet of managing organ-specific manifestations during pregnancy is to have the disease under good control on medications compatible with pregnancy for several months prior to conception (Table 5.2). However, even the best-made plans go awry and at times the clinician may be faced with complicated organ system flares during pregnancy that require adjustments to medications. When disease is life- or organ-threatening, medication choice needs to be liberalized in order to get the disease under control as quickly as possible. In this chapter, we will discuss some of the more common complicated organ-specific flares during pregnancy and their management.

Box 5.1 Physiological and laboratory changes of pregnancy that impact monitoring of rheumatological disease

---

Physiological
Muscle pain
Joint pain
Fatigue
Back pain
Oedema

Laboratory
Physiological anaemia
Elevated ESR
Increased synthesis of complement components
Increase in white blood cell count
Decrease in uric acid

Case 1: Autoimmune skin disease

A 33-year-old woman who has a history of severe subacute cutaneous lupus presents for pre-pregnancy counselling. Her skin disease is currently controlled with hydroxychloroquine 200 mg twice a day and mycophenolate mofetil (MMF) 1000 mg twice daily. In the past, when immunosuppression has been discontinued, she developed significant skin lesions over her trunk and arms that become superinfected. In anticipation of pregnancy, the treatment plan was to discontinue the MMF and transition the patient to azathioprine. However, testing revealed that the patient had a low level of thiopurine S-methyltransferase (TPMT) enzyme activity, rendering her a poor metabolizer of and therefore not a candidate for this medication as she is at risk for bone marrow suppression. She is eager to have a pre-pregnancy plan in place.

Table 5.1 Differentiating connective tissue disease/SLE flare from pre-eclampsia/HELLP

Clinical finding	CTD/SLE flare	Pre-eclampsia
Timing	All three trimesters	Rare before 20 weeks, most often after 34 weeks
Hypertension	+/−	+++
Oedema	+	+++
Proteinuria	++	+++
Thrombocytopenia	++	+++
Liver function tests	Unchanged or decreased	++
Rising dsDNA antibody titre	++	−
Complement levels	Low or falling	Normal or high

Table 5.2 Medications and pregnancy

Medication	Comment
Minimal Risk	
Hydroxychloroquine	
Sulfasalazine	
Azathioprine/6-mercaptopurine	Check TPMT
Baby aspirin	
Some Risk	
NSAIDs	Stop in the 3rd trimester—risk of premature closure
Glucocorticoids—keep low	ductus arteriosus
Tumour necrosis factor	Minimize dose to avoid diabetes, hypertension, pre-
Intravenous immune globulin	term premature rupture of membranes (PPROM),
Ciclosporin	small-for-gestational-age (SGA)
Tacrolimus	Consider discontinuation in the 3rd trimester for
	monoclonal antibodies with high placenta passage
Moderate to High Risk	
Cyclophosphamide	Consider use late 2nd or 3rd trimester in life-threatening
Rituximab	conditions
Methotrexate	Should be discontinued—consider use in life-threatening
Mycophenolate mofetil	conditions
Leflunomide	Stop medication 1–3 months prior to conception
	Stop medication 6 weeks prior to conception
	Cholestyramine washout until levels are undetectable
Use until Conception	
Belimumab	IgG based therapies do not cross the placenta in detectable
Abatacept	amounts until the 12th week of gestation
Actemra	
Anakinra	
Ustekinumab	
Secukinumab	
No data	
Tofacitinib	
Baracitinib	

Case discussion

Skin disease in SLE can be either a part of the systemic disease or can occur in isolation. The two most common skin entities seen clinically are discoid lupus erythematosus (DLE) and subacute cutaneous lupus erythematosus (SCLE). Discoid lesions occur predominantly on the face and on the scalp and can lead to scarring and depigmentation. SCLE lesions in general occur in photo-exposed areas and present as either psoriaform or annular lesions. With severe flares, involvement can be extensive and superinfection of lesions can occur. Treatment includes sun avoidance, antimalarials, topical and systemic steroids. In more severe cases, systemic anti-metabolites such as methotrexate and immunosuppression such as ciclosporin, azathioprine, and tacrolimus may be used.

Careful pregnancy planning in women with SLE can decrease flare risk. Patients with a prior history of renal disease, active disease in the 6 months preceding pregnancy, and primigravidas are the most likely to flare. In general, organ-specific disease activity in the 6 months prior to pregnancy can predict organ-specific flare during pregnancy. An important component of pre-pregnancy care in SLE patients is transitioning patients to medications compatible with pregnancy and observing patients for a period of time on these medications. In the aforementioned case, MMF is teratogenic and needs to be discontinued. As the patient requires immunosuppression in order to control her skin disease, she needs to be transitioned to another medication that is compatible with pregnancy. There is ample experience using azathioprine during pregnancy with tens of thousands of transplant patients being treated with this medication during pregnancy with no increased risk of congenital anomalies in offspring exposed to this medication in utero. In general, for SLE patients, this would be the first choice for immunosuppression in a pregnant patient. Nonetheless, patients who lack adequate TPMT enzyme activity are not candidates for this therapy. Another option for management in this patient would be transitioning her to oral tacrolimus, an immunosuppressive agent that is compatible with pregnancy. In this case, the patient should have her MMF stopped. Tacrolimus should be initiated and the patient should be observed for several months prior to attempting pregnancy to make sure that she does not experience any disease flare.

Case 2: Inflammatory arthritis during pregnancy

A 27-year-old previously healthy medicine resident is 21 weeks pregnant with her first pregnancy. She presents with 3–4 months of progressive deep buttock pain and low back stiffness in the mornings. It has now worsened to the point where it is interfering with her ability to function at work. Acetaminophen has not helped her symptoms and she has avoided non-steroidal anti-inflammatory drugs (NSAIDs) during her pregnancy. She denies any peripheral arthritis or any other symptoms outside of fatigue. She had her level II ultrasound at gestational week 20 that was without any abnormalities. On physical examination, she has markedly reduced forward flexion, beyond what would be expected with a 21-week pregnancy. Blood testing showed an ESR of 62 and a slightly elevated CRP but otherwise normal results. Magnetic resonance imaging (MRI) of her hips and pelvis shows acute inflammation of and early erosive changes in both sacroiliac joints. She asks what she should do next.

Case discussion

This is a young woman with early acute bilateral sacroiliitis that developed during an otherwise uncomplicated pregnancy. Because seronegative spondyloarthropathies are much less common among women of childbearing age, there are little data regarding the effects of underlying disease on pregnancy outcomes. However, we can extrapolate from other inflammatory arthritides that systemic inflammation may complicate pregnancy and may impair full foetal growth and lead to parturition at an earlier gestational age. The elevated ESR is difficult to interpret as it rises significantly—in general up to a level of 40—during healthy pregnancies; however, a level of 63 is higher than expected. The CRP, on the other hand, may be more reflective of systemic elevation due to increased inflammation outside of pregnancy. The patient is symptomatic, suffering increasing difficulty with vocational activities, and her reduced mobility may have adverse long-term consequences. The goal in this case would be to achieve both rapid and effective reduction of systemic inflammation and improved function for the remaining 18–19 weeks of pregnancy. Therefore, treatment is recommended.

The most common forms of autoimmune or inflammatory arthritis affecting women of childbearing age are in the setting of SLE, rheumatoid arthritis, and the seronegative spondyloarthropathies. The risks of adverse pregnancy outcomes among women with uncontrolled inflammatory arthritis have been well described in many cohorts and therefore control of disease is paramount in caring for women during their pregnancies. In cases where the diagnosis has been made prior to pregnancy, all attempts should be made to assure disease quiescence on medications known to be compatible with pregnancy. Medications used for inflammatory arthritis with known teratogenic potential or insufficient pregnancy experience should be stopped prior to conception (methotrexate, leflunomide, new small molecule biologics) and the patient should be followed for several months on medications that can be continued throughout pregnancy (low-dose steroids, hydroxychloroquine, sulfasalazine, azathioprine, tumour necrosis factor (TNF) inhibitors) to ensure that the underlying disease can be well controlled on the new medicine regime and necessary adjustments can be made. In cases of pregnancy occurring while the woman is taking potentially teratogenic medications, these should be discontinued immediately and patients should be referred to a maternal-foetal medicine specialist for consultation. Women on leflunomide who are anticipating pregnancy or who inadvertently become pregnant should receive cholestyramine until blood levels are undetectable (see Chapter 3.1).

In general, the therapy choices for autoimmune arthritis during pregnancy should mirror the most optimal choices for the non-pregnant person. Data gathered from non-pregnant populations consistently demonstrates a lack of efficacy of methotrexate and sulfasalazine for axial disease; corticosteroids also have limited efficacy. Moreover, methotrexate is contraindicated during pregnancy although sulfasalazine is not. In the aforementioned case, TNF inhibitors (TNFi) are the most effective treatments for active sacroiliitis and spondylitis. After confirmation of a negative tuberculosis testing, she should be started on a TNFi with low placenta passage as monotherapy. While most TNFi do cross the placenta by week 16 of gestation, with levels that supersede maternal levels by 40 weeks, there is little indication that elevated levels in neonates contribute to unacceptable infection risks in the newborn. However, if the patient is prescribed a TNFi during pregnancy, then she should be advised to have her newborn avoid live vaccines (Bacille–Calmette Guérin (BCG) and rotavirus) for the first 6 months of life. She may also elect to discontinue therapy in the mid-3rd trimester out of concern for infection risk, but this must be weighed against the risk of flare of axial disease around the time of delivery.

This approach is also applicable to the management of rheumatoid arthritis and psoriatic arthritis during pregnancy. Milder cases of rheumatoid arthritis may be managed with non-biological options including hydroxychloroquine and/or sulfasalazine. More severe disease can be managed with TNFi. In cases of inflammatory arthritis related to SLE, hydroxychloroquine and azathioprine may be among the most effective options that can be continued throughout pregnancy.

Corticosteroids should be reserved for acute exacerbations of disease activity during pregnancy that require immediate treatment. As in non-pregnant patients, the lowest dose of steroids should be used to control disease activity. Upon initiation of steroids, steroid sparing agents should be discussed with the patient. For patients who are on long-term, stable, low-dose corticosteroids, they should be maintained for the duration of pregnancy on the dose that has been used to maintain control, as any attempts to taper may increase risk of flare. However, the institution of low-dose corticosteroids in an otherwise stable patient for the sole purposes of reducing risk of flare during pregnancy has not been shown to improve pregnancy outcomes.

Case 3: Haematological disorders during pregnancy

A 31-year-old woman with SLE has successfully conceived her second pregnancy. She has a 3-year-old healthy child, and in anticipation of pregnancy has achieved good control of her underlying disease with hydroxychloroquine and prednisone 5 mg daily. Past SLE manifestations included malar rash, inflammatory arthritis, thrombocytopenia, and leukopenia, and currently she has only a mild malar rash. Pre-conception platelet count has been stable at 90,000. Her pregnancy is uneventful and she returns to clinic for routine follow-up at week 29. Platelet count at that visit has fallen to 30,000. Prednisone is increased to 20 mg daily. One week later, her platelet count has fallen to 22,000 and she has noticed increased bruising on her legs and forearms. After a long discussion with the patient and her partner, prednisone is immediately increased to 60 mg daily and a course of rituximab is planned (1 gram IV day 1 and day 14). Platelet count increases to 82,000. Prednisone is tapered back to 20 mg daily and platelets remain stable above 70,000 for the remainder of pregnancy.

Case discussion

Pregnancy itself is accompanied by an increase in white blood cell count *but* a mild dilutional decrease in the haematocrit and platelet count. The latter are a consequence of the increased plasma volume that occurs in the early weeks of pregnancy and do not require any intervention aside from following a complete blood count (CBC) every trimester. In cases where a pregnant woman has a history of immune thrombocytopenia or haemolytic anaemia or develops symptoms suggestive of active haematological disease, monitoring may need to be more frequent and intervention may be warranted. The decision to treat autoimmune cytopenias in pregnant women depends on the degree of anaemia or thrombocytopenia as well as the rapidity of the drop. Mild, asymptomatic cytopenias, even if representative of active peripheral destruction, may not necessarily need intervention if the counts stay in a reasonable range: platelet count above 60,000–70,000 and haemoglobin above 9 or 9.5. Counts below these begin to place the patient and the pregnancy at risk. For example, platelet counts below 20,000 or 25,000 can cause spontaneous haemorrhage, even life-threatening cerebral haemorrhage. In cases of mild to moderate autoimmune haemolytic anaemia or thrombocytopenia, corticosteroids have a rapid onset of action and are often effective. Azathioprine may provide additional long-term control, allowing for reduction or taper of steroids. However, in cases of severe life-threatening cytopenias, rituximab is the intervention of choice. It has a relatively short time to onset of action, and its intermittent dosing schedule of 6-month intervals (if needed) makes it a potentially good option where severe disease occurs during an established pregnancy. As an IgG1 kappa constructed monoclonal antibody, rituximab requires active transport across the placenta into foetal circulation that does not begin until week 16. Therefore, in the peri-conception period or 1st trimester of pregnancy, active drug will not reach the foetal circulation and mothers can be treated without fear of foetal exposure. After 16 weeks' gestation, foetal levels of rituximab increase in concentration, thus raising concerns for adverse effects of foetal exposure. Reassuringly, review of the rituximab global safety database of rituximab given during the 2nd or 3rd trimester of established pregnancy in order to treat life-threatening maternal diseases did not reveal undue risk of neonatal compromise or infection. A few infants had mild cytopenias or absent peripheral B cells at birth, but this was not related to increased risk of infection. Therefore, in cases of severe or life-threatening autoimmune haematological manifestations during pregnancy, at whatever stage they occur, rituximab may be a reasonable option to help restore blood cell counts to acceptable levels and minimize the high-dose corticosteroids that may otherwise be required for extended periods of time until pregnancy is completed. Currently, there is no need for CBC monitoring of the newborn unless symptoms of infection, anaemia, or bleeding are present. In rare cases where rituximab therapy is ineffective, other salvage therapies may include intravenous immunoglobulin infusion, plasma exchange, or splenectomy in the setting of peri-operative red blood cell or platelet transfusion.

Case 4: Diffuse alveolar haemorrhage

A 27-year-old woman with a history of SLE (positive serologies, skin disease, arthritis, and the presence of anti-phospholipid antibodies) presents to the emergency room with haemoptysis for 3 days during her 23rd week of pregnancy. Radiographic evaluation reveals diffuse pulmonary infiltrates and bronchoalveolar lavage confirms pulmonary haemorrhage. She is transferred to the medical intensive care unit (ICU) for further management.

Case discussion

Diffuse alveolar haemorrhage (DAH) is one of the most challenging presentations in rheumatology. This clinical entity can be seen in patients with SLE, mixed connective tissue disease, rheumatoid arthritis, antiphospholipid syndrome, small vessel vasculitis such as immunoglobulin A (IgA) vasculopathy, cryoglobulinaemia, and granulomatosis with polyangiitis. Upwards of 50% of patients with DAH die. Pregnancy can further complicate management, thus prompt recognition and treatment of this disorder are imperative. High-dose steroids such as a gram of solumedrol a day are the first line of therapy. Plasma exchange, often used in this dire clinical presentation, is compatible with pregnancy, although fluid shifts need to be carefully monitored. Two other medications are often used to manage this disorder in the non-pregnant case. Rituximab is also considered standard of care; however, it is generally recommended to discontinue this medication at the time of conception (see previous discussion). The presentation of DAH is life threatening and aggressive therapy is indicated, thus this is another scenario in which rituximab can be considered. Similarly, while cyclophosphamide is contraindicated during pregnancy this agent can be considered if the patient does not appear to respond to other therapies such as pulse steroids and plasma exchange. After initial immunosuppression and stabilization, an immunosuppressive agent that is compatible with pregnancy such as azathioprine should be initiated.

Other pulmonary manifestations of rheumatological diseases are common. Pleuritis is seen most frequently and in general can be treated with low-dose steroids and colchicine, both of which are compatible with pregnancy. All SLE patients should be counselled to stay on hydroxychloroquine; this is often an effective agent to control pleuritis. Pneumonitis can also be a presentation of rheumatic diseases. Many patients with pneumonitis are being treated with low-dose steroids and immunosuppressive therapy: the same tenets for immunosuppressive agents compatible with pregnancy that were discussed previously can be applied here.

Case 5: Cardiac disease

A 33-year-old woman with a 1-year history of SLE (+ antinuclear antibody (ANA), double-stranded DNA (dsDNA), mild lymphopenia, arthritis, and low complements well controlled on hydroxychloroquine monotherapy) presents to the emergency room at 19 weeks gestational age with a 2-day history of shortness of breath, inspiratory chest pain, and worsening arthritis. Physical examination was notable for clear breath sounds, tachycardia, tachypnea, and muffled heart sounds. She had active synovitis in both wrists and scattered metacarpophalangeal (MCP) joints. In the emergency room, she underwent a computed tomography (CT) angiogram of the pulmonary arteries, which was negative for a pulmonary embolus. Echocardiogram demonstrated a moderate to large pericardial effusion without tamponade physiology. Ultrasonographic evaluation of the foetus was unremarkable. She was admitted to the hospital for further evaluation and management. Rheumatology consultation diagnosed a moderate to severe lupus flare and she was immediately treated with 1,000 mg of intravenous methylprednisolone daily for 3 days with significant improvement in her symptoms. She was discharged on 60 mg prednisone daily and continuation of hydroxychloroquine. One week post discharge she was evaluated in rheumatology and found to be stable. In attempts to reduce the overall steroid burden, azathioprine was added to her regimen and prednisone was decreased to 40 mg daily. Within a week, her dyspnea and pleuritic chest pain returned. Prednisone was increased to 80 mg daily. Repeated echocardiograms showed very slow resolution of the effusion, and prednisone was kept at 60 mg daily. After 8 weeks, her effusion was minimal and she was able to tolerate a slow wean of prednisone to 20 mg daily over the next 6 weeks. Foetal growth was normal.

At 35 weeks, she had spontaneous rupture of membranes followed by increase in blood pressure and new onset proteinuria concerning for pre-eclampsia. She underwent emergency Caesarean delivery at 35 weeks to deliver a female infant weighting 5 lb, 10 oz. The infant was otherwise healthy.

Case discussion

Fortunately, cardiac disease is relatively uncommon with most systemic rheumatic diseases, and most often presents as pericarditis in patients with SLE or as myocarditis in patients with eosinophilic granulomatosus with polyangiitis (Churg–Strauss syndrome). These manifestations can be very symptomatic and even risk optimal cardiac function and often necessitate urgent and aggressive therapy. This is especially true for the pregnant patient who must maintain adequate cardiac output to support a pregnancy. Therefore, corticosteroids are usually the first line of therapy to treat active inflammatory cardiac disease because of their rapid onset of action and ability to titrate to disease activity. Non-fluorinated corticosteroids (such as methylprednisone and prednisone) are largely inactivated by the placenta, so reduced levels reach foetal circulation. Although there are concerns with use of higher doses of corticosteroids during pregnancy due to increased risks of spontaneous rupture of membranes and prematurity, risks of active cardiac disease and cardiac compromise must outweigh these concerns. In this case, high doses of steroids were successful in reducing symptoms quite rapidly, but they returned with early taper of prednisone before the immunosuppressive effects of azathioprine were established. In general, after high-dose steroids are initiated and disease is controlled, a steroid-sparing immunosuppressant medication that is compatible with pregnancy should be initiated as soon as possible to allow for steroid taper. Steroid-sparing agents include azathioprine, colchicine, and even rituximab may be considered for severe, refractory disease. Cyclophosphamide may be considered in the 2nd or 3rd trimester as salvage therapy in life-threatening cases.

Because pregnancy itself is a pro-thrombotic condition, pulmonary embolism must be considered in every case of moderate to severe chest pain or dyspnea as anticoagulation may be critical in preventing maternal morbidity and mortality from venous thromboembolism. In pregnant women with a moderate to high pre-test probability of pulmonary embolism, CT angiography in addition to D-dimer testing and lower limb ultrasonography can safely exclude venous thromboembolism.

Case 6: Cerebral disease

A 27-year-old previously healthy woman presents during her 29th week of pregnancy with right-sided weakness and an expressive aphasia. MRA reveals beading in the left-middle cerebral artery that is consistent with central nervous system (CNS) vasculitis. The patients ESR is 110 and her CRP is 43. History and physical examination other than the findings previously described are unremarkable. Autoantibody work-up is negative. The diagnosis of isolated CNS vasculitis is made.

Case discussion

CNS vasculitis is a rare entity that either occurs in the setting of SLE and vasculitis but more commonly presents as an isolated disorder. There are focal neurological findings with elevations of inflammatory markers and classic findings of beading on CNS vessel imaging. Ideally, diagnosis is confirmed with leptomeningeal biopsy but at times that is not feasible. This condition carries high morbidity for the patients. Initial therapy should be with high-dose glucocorticoid pulse. However, this is usually inadequate to ensure disease control. This case presents a clinical dilemma as to the next line of therapy; recommendations are to avoid cyclophosphamide and rituximab during pregnancy if possible. However, as most of organogenesis has occurred and given the morbidity of this presentation, cyclophosphamide therapy can be considered. If the pregnancy were in the 3rd trimester, this medication could be considered. While rituximab will start to cross the placenta after 12 weeks of gestation, limited data do not suggest long-term harm to the foetus if used after this time. For this particular case, we would recommend cyclophosphamide therapy dosing and then initiation of azathioprine therapy for maintenance.

Key messages

- Rheumatic diseases are challenging to manage during pregnancy because disease flares are unpredictable and not all medications can be continued during pregnancy (see Chapter 3.1).
- Making certain that underlying disease is well controlled at the time of conception on medications compatible with pregnancy is the best way to ensure a good pregnancy outcome for the mother and the developing foetus.
- Mild disease flares such as mild skin disease, minimal thrombocytopenia, and mild joint symptoms can be managed by either background medications or low doses of steroids.
- Severe disease flares such as pulmonary haemorrhage and cerebritis requires high-dose steroids and immunosuppressive therapy. In these circumstances, the clinician may need to make the difficult choice of using medications that are contraindicated during pregnancy in order to ensure maternal recovery.

Further reading

1. Leatherwood C, Bermas BL. Drugs and pregnancy In: *Rheumatology*, seventh edition. Hochberg MC, Silman AJ, Smolen JS, Weinblatt ME, Weisman MH (eds). St. Louis, MO: Mosby; 2017.
2. Smith CJF, Bandoli G, Kavanaugh A, Chambers CD. Birth outcomes and disease activity during pregnancy in a prospective cohort of women with psoriatic arthritis and ankylosing spondylitis. *Arthritis Care Res*. 2019; doi: 10.1002/acr.23924. [Epub ahead of print]
3. Nelson-Piercy C, Argarwal S, Lams B. Lesson of the month: Selective use of cyclophosphamide in pregnancy for severe autoimmune respiratory disease. *Thorax*. 2016;71:667–8.

4. de Man YA, Hazes JM, van der Heide H, Willemsen SP, de Groot CJ, Steegers EA, Dolhain RJ. Association of higher rheumatoid arthritis disease activity during pregnancy with lower birth weight: Results of a national prospective study. *Arthritis Rheum*. 2009;60:3196–206.
5. Singh P, Dhooria A, Rathi M, Agarwal R, Sharma K, Dhir V, et al. Successful treatment outcomes in pregnant patients with ANCA-associated vasculitides: A systematic review of the literature. *Int J Rheum Dis*. 2018;21:1734–40.

SECTION VI
OBSTETRIC COMPLICATIONS IN WOMEN WITH AUTOIMMUNE DISEASES

6

Pregnancy and obstetric complications in women with autoimmune diseases

D. Ware Branch

Selected aspects of prenatal care and normal pregnancy physiology

Early gestation (conception through 9 weeks)

Identifying pregnancy: for most women, pregnancy is suspected when the symptoms of early pregnancy develop—these include breast soreness or tenderness, fatigue, nausea, and missed menses. Human chorionic gonadotropin (hCG) is first detectable using sensitive tests in the urine and blood of pregnant women 8–10 days after conception (day 22–24 of a 28-day menstrual cycle). Concentrations of hCG rise rapidly in early pregnancy, peak at 9–10 weeks, and decline thereafter to a nadir at 20 weeks.

Dating the pregnancy: human pregnancy duration averages 280 days from the 1st day of the last menstrual period. The use of the 1st day of the last menstrual period to mark the 'beginning' of pregnancy is one of historical convention, and it is customary for obstetricians to 'date' pregnancy in terms of weeks and days from the beginning of the last menstrual period rather that from conception. Since conception occurs about 2 weeks from the 1st day of the last menstrual period (in an average 28-day menstrual cycle), the conventional obstetric gestational age includes 14 days during which the woman was not pregnant. Thus, a pregnancy of 10 'weeks of gestation' is actually 8 weeks post-conception. Current obstetric practice includes confirming the gestational age of the pregnancy via foetal ultrasound using standard biometric measurements of the crown–rump length in early pregnancy or a mathematically modelled composite of the measurements of the foetal head, abdomen, and femur in later pregnancy. Generally, and especially if the menstrual dates are uncertain, the ultrasound-determined dates trump menstrual dates when they differ by more than more than 5 days <9 weeks of gestation, more than 7 days, 9–15[6] weeks of gestation, or more than 10 days, 16–21[6] weeks of gestation. Because foetal size varies considerably as pregnancy advances, measurement of the foetal parameters is a less reliable tool for estimation of gestational age past the mid-2nd trimester and especially in the 3rd trimester.

Initial prenatal visits and laboratory tests: the initial prenatal encounter typically includes a history and physical examination and if available standard 'prenatal labs', including a complete blood count (CBC), human immunodeficiency virus (HIV), and hepatitis (i.e. hepatitis B surface antigen (HBSAg)) screening, and ABO, and Rh blood typing with anti-erythrocyte antibody screening. Women with rheumatic diseases may also have tests for urine protein-to-creatinine ratio, complete metabolic panel, antiphospholipid antibodies, and anti-Sjögren's-syndrome-related antigen A (anti-SSA/SSB) antibodies (Table 6.1). In many locales, it is common practice to obtain a 1st or early 2nd trimester foetal ultrasound to firmly establish the gestational age and due date. Within the 1st trimester, the new prenatal patient should be apprised of the risks of foetal genetic conditions such as Down's syndrome or autosomal recessive diseases and offered screening tests for these conditions. With regard to foetal chromosomal aneuploidy, cell-free foetal deoxyribonucleic acid (DNA) screening has become a very popular choice.

Embryonic development: fertilization of the ovum occurs in the fallopian tube, and the zygote migrates into the uterus over the course of 5–6 days. The rapidly dividing cells of the zygote form a fluid-filled structure known as the blastocyst with external and internal cellular components. The external cells are destined to interact with the uterine endometrium and form the trophoblastic (placental) tissue, while a separate group of cells form the inner cell mass, destined to form the embryo and enclosing membrane structures. The blastocyst implants into the endometrial lining (endometrium) to become completely interstitial between 6 and 12 days (on average 9 days) post-conception. The trophoblastic cells of the blastocyst in contact with the decidualized endometrium form an invasive, multinucleated syncytium, the syncytiotrophoblast, an invasive and secretory tissue distinct from more proximal, single-cell cytotrophoblastic tissue. After implantation, the syncytiotrophoblast just under the forming embryo and amniotic cavity thickens and then forms a matrix of trabeculae and vacuolar spaces, precursors to the placental villi and intervillous spaces. About the 12th day after conception, the more internal cytotrophoblastic cells migrate to the distal tips of the trabeculae and spread laterally to form a new, surrounding cytotrophoblastic layer, or 'shell'. In the third week after conception, extraembryonic mesodermal cells and haemangioblasts invade the more proximal areas of the trabeculae to form foetal villous vasculature.

Pluripotent cells of the inner cell mass give rise to the embryo in a remarkably complex process that is beyond the context of this review. Briefly, the inner cell mass differentiates into a two-cell layer structure, called the germ disc, initially comprised of an epiblastic layer and endodermal layer. The latter further differentiates into extraembryonic endoderm, which forms the yolk sac, and visceral endoderm that ultimately gives rise to embryonic endoderm and mesodermal tissues. Subsequent development involves cellular migration and differentiation in a process known as gastrulation, a process that results in the formation of germ layers (endoderm, mesoderm, and ectoderm) and the necessary embryonic axes (dorsoventral, craniocaudal, and left-right). Gastrulation results in critical alterations of cellular interactions that, in turn, allow for the formation of a neural tube (neurulation) and organogenesis. It is during this period of development that embryonic teratogens, such as warfarin, act to result in maldevelopment leading to birth defects or syndromic features. By the 8th post-conception week (10th gestational week), all major organs are formed, though further development and refinement are ongoing processes. Though semantic in nature, obstetricians generally regard the period from

Table 6.1 Recommended practices in pregnancies of women with systemic lupus erythematosus (SLE), antiphospholipid syndrome (APS), and rheumatoid arthritis (RA)

Assessment/Test	Pre-con-ception	1st trimester	18–20 weeks	22–24 weeks	26–28 weeks	30–32 weeks	32–34 weeks	36–38 weeks
SLE								
Adjustments of drug therapy to minimize risks[1]	X							
Laboratory assessments								
Antiphospholipid antibodies	X							
CBC with platelets	X	X						
Renal function and protein excretion	X	X						
Screen for gestational diabetes[1]			X		X	X		
Obstetric ultrasound for foetal growth and amniotic fluid volume			X	X	X	X	X	X
Foetal surveillance tests[2]			X			X---------------------------------		
APS								
Adjustments of drug therapy to minimize risks	X	X[3]						
Laboratory assessments								
CBC with platelets	X	X						
Assessment of anticoagulation[4]		X	X		X		X	

(continued)

Table 6.1 Continued

Assessment/Test	Pre-con-ception	1st trimester	18–20 weeks	22–24 weeks	26–28 weeks	30–32 weeks	32–34 weeks	36–38 weeks
Obstetric ultrasound for foetal growth and amniotic fluid volume			X	X	X	X	X	X
Foetal surveillance tests[2]						X------		------
RA								
Adjustments of drug therapy to minimize risks	X							
Obstetric ultrasound for foetal growth and amniotic fluid volume			X		X[5]	X	X	
Foetal surveillance tests[2]						X[5]------		------
CBC—complete blood count								

[1] Routine gestational diabetes screening is performed at 24–28 weeks of gestation in otherwise low-risk patients. However, for women on chronic glucocorticoids, earlier and more frequent screening is recommended.

[2] May include non-stress tests, amniotic fluid volume assessment, biophysical profiles, uterine and/or foetal vascular Doppler assessment, or a combination of these. Foetal surveillance testing is typically performed on a twice weekly basis, though practices may vary according to the degree of clinical concern.

[3] If the patient is on warfarin, it should be discontinued before 6 weeks' gestation to avoid warfarin embryopathy.

[4] For women in whom full anticoagulation is the goal. Note that there is considerable variation in practice as to how often assessment of anticoagulation status is done.

[5] The clinical utility of serial obstetric ultrasound to assess foetal growth and amniotic fluid volume in women with RA and an otherwise uncomplicated pregnancy is uncertain.

10 gestational weeks forward as the 'foetal' period, while the period of development leading up to this is the 'embryonic' period.

During the first 10 weeks of gestation, the lacunae of the forming placenta are filled with clear fluid, without the presence of a genuine relationship between maternal and embryonic circulations. Thus, during this period, gas and nutrient exchange with the embryonic structures is of a passive nature, with intervillous space oxygen concentrations being <20 mm Hg. In the meantime, the terminal portions of the uterine arteries that penetrate into the decidualized endometrium, known as spiral arterioles, have undergone remarkable alteration, with replacement of vascular wall smooth muscle and elastic fibres with fibrinoid resulting in a dilated, non-muscular terminal arteriolar structure. Within the first few weeks of pregnancy, migrating extravillous cytotrophoblastic cells associate with the altered terminal spiral arterioles. Some of these cells invade the vascular lumina and replace the endothelial cells therein, temporarily occluding the vessels. Other extravillous cytotrophoblast cells pass through the endometrium into the inner third of the myometrium and form multinucleated giant cells. In association with this, further dilation of the terminal spiral arteries occurs such that the terminal arteriolar structure now appears somewhat funnel shaped. Other important changes in the maternal vasculature have been in play. The more distal segments of the spiral arteries also dilate under the influence of pregnancy-related hormones, and the overall maternal blood flow to the uterus begins to increase considerably.

Maternal physiology: for the majority of pregnant women, the embryonic period (through the 9th week of gestation) is marked by symptoms of early pregnancy, including breast tenderness, nausea, easy fatigability, and other physical concerns. Due to some of these symptoms, maternal weight gain in early pregnancy may be limited, and some women lose a small amount of weight. A number of dramatic physiological changes occur in early pregnancy. An increase in maternal plasma volume begins by about 6 weeks of gestation. The maternal cardiac ventricular mass increases, and maternal cardiac output increases by approximately 15–20% by as early as 8 weeks of gestation due largely to increased stroke volume, but also to an early increase in heart rate. Systemic vascular resistance decreases from 5 weeks of gestation forward. An increase in minute ventilation due to an increase in tidal volume results in a decrease in maternal partial pressure of arterial carbon dioxide ($PaCO_2$) and a mild respiratory alkalosis. Maternal respiratory rate is not increased, though many pregnant women notice a sense of breathlessness intermittently during pregnancy. Renal plasma flow also increases beginning in early pregnancy, and this in combination with alterations in pre- and post-glomerular vasodilation result in the glomerular filtration rate (GFR) approaching 50% above non-pregnant rates by 10 weeks of gestation.

Mid-gestation (10 weeks through 27 weeks)

Ongoing prenatal care: in otherwise healthy pregnant women, periodic prenatal visits are used to assess the foetal and maternal status. The growth of the uterus is assessed by palpation and fundal height measurement (done after 20 weeks). Foetal heart rate is assessed via Doppler or ultrasound visualization. Maternal blood pressure is checked, and the maternal urine is screened for evidence of infection and proteinuria using urine dipsticks. These assessments are particularly important in women with autoimmune diseases that predispose to gestational hypertensive disease (Table 6.1). After 20–22 weeks, the mother is also questioned routinely regarding the presence of foetal movement.

Depending on the country, women are offered routine ultrasound scans. Some countries offer a routine 12-week ultrasound scan as part of the so-called 'triple test'. At approximately 20 weeks, a mid-trimester obstetric ultrasound examination of the foetus is obtained to confirm the expected gestational age and to assess the foetal anatomy by way of well-established, standardized views of numerous foetal structures, such as the foetal heart, intracranial contents, and abdominal wall. A normal foetal anatomic survey excludes a majority of serious foetal anomalies. In women at risk for foetal growth restriction, e.g. those with antiphospholipid syndrome (APS), ultrasound assessment of foetal growth and amniotic fluid volume can be offered more often, i.e. several weeks after 18–20 weeks of gestation (Table 6.1).

Screening for gestational diabetes mellitus between 24 and 28 weeks of gestation is routine and should be done somewhat earlier in pregnancy in women at higher risk for gestational diabetes, such as obese women or those on glucocorticoids (Table 6.1).

Foetal development: establishment of the human haemochorial placental circulation starts at 10–12 weeks of gestation when the cellular occlusion of terminal spiral arterioles begins to clear, allowing maternal blood to enter the intervillous space and bathe the foetal villi; as result, the oxygen tension in the intervillous space rises. Maturation of the foetal villi and foetal production of capable (non-nucleated) erythrocytes complete the requirements for a true placental circulation. The intervillous circulation is of relatively high volume and low velocity, such that the pressure within the intervillous space is relatively low, lower than that in the foetal villous vasculature. The net result is that oxygenated maternal blood can enter the intervillous space and bathe the delicate foetal villi without damaging or collapsing them.

By the early 2nd trimester, the exocoelomic cavity shrinks, with the amnion then fusing with the chorion, leaving the amniotic fluid as the sole fluid surrounding the foetus. This fluid results from foetal renal and pulmonary fluid production; it 'circulates' as a result of foetal swallowing and membrane resorption. Amniotic fluid is required for normal foetal development, and it likely serves several major roles, including bacteriostasis, cushioning, and accommodation of spatial dynamics. During mid-pregnancy, the amniotic fluid volume increases to reach an average volume of 700 mL by 27 weeks.

Expressed as a percentage of increased weight per week, the rate of foetal growth is highest in the first 10–12 weeks of pregnancy and declines thereafter. However, expressed as weight gain per day or week, e.g. grams of weight gained per day, foetal growth proceeds at a modest rate during the first half of pregnancy, reaching about 10 grams per day by 20 weeks, and demonstrates the most rapid growth beginning about 22–24 weeks of gestation. Foetal growth during this period, and extending into the 3rd trimester, is a result of cellular hyperplasia and cellular hypertrophy.

Maternal physiology: maternal plasma volume and red cell mass continue to increase. Maternal cardiac stroke volume reaches its maximum by 20 weeks of gestation and maintains through the 2nd trimester in conjunction with an increase in maternal heart rate. The decrease in systemic vascular resistance is primarily responsible for a fall in systolic and diastolic blood pressures that reach a nadir about 10 mm Hg lower than in the non-pregnant state in the mid-trimester. An increase in minute ventilation due to an increase in tidal volume results in a decrease in maternal $PaCO_2$ and a mild respiratory alkalosis. Maternal respiratory rate is not increased, though many pregnant women notice a sense of breathlessness intermittently during pregnancy. Renal plasma flow is maximal by 20–24 weeks of gestation, and GFR is moderately increased compared to the non-pregnant state.

3rd trimester (28 weeks through delivery)

Ongoing prenatal care: prenatal visits every 2 weeks may be offered, though more frequent visits may be warranted in women with rheumatic diseases (Table 6.1). It is particularly important to assess maternal blood pressure and other potential markers of gestational hypertensive diseases. Concern about foetal growth and the possibility of foetal growth restriction may require ultrasound evaluation.

Pregnancies complicated by rheumatic diseases such as systemic lupus or APS are not only monitored periodically for evidence of foetal growth restriction, but also are managed in the 3rd trimester with enhanced foetal assessment because of the risk of placental insufficiency (Table 6.1). The most common foetal surveillance tests in routine use are the non-stress test (NST), assessment of amniotic fluid volume as an index (AFI), and the biophysical profile test (BPP). The NST test is usually done once or twice weekly and employs a Doppler monitoring system to record a continuous foetal heart rate tracing. The presence of foetal heart accelerations with foetal movement are indicative of a neurologically intact brainstem-cardiac circuitry; the absence of these raises concern for severe impairment in maternal-placental circulation and severe foetal hypoxaemia. Amniotic fluid volume is assessed using ultrasound, with AFI normally in excess of 5 cm by 4-quadrant measurement or 2 cm as the deepest vertical pocket; lower measurements are concerning for worsening maternal-placental circulation.

Analysis of in utero vascular Doppler velocimetry waveforms has been added to foetal surveillance testing for selected patients, particularly those with foetal growth restriction. The most commonly used foetal vascular Doppler assessment is measurement of resistance to flow in the umbilical arteries, with evidence of increasing resistance to flow reflective of worsening maternal-placental circulation and worsening oxygenation of the foetus.

Foetal development: The rate of foetal growth in terms of weight gain per week peaks at approximately 250 grams per week at 32–34 weeks of gestation. The rate of foetal growth declines thereafter to reach about 100 grams per week at 39–40 weeks. Amniotic fluid volume is greatest at 34 weeks of gestation (about 800 mL) and declines to about 600 mL at 40 weeks.

Maternal physiology: A disproportionate increase in plasma volume relative to red cell mass results in a physiological 'anaemia' of pregnancy by the middle of the 3rd trimester. Maternal cardiac stroke volume declines a bit in the late-3rd trimester, though maternal heart rate is maximal (about 85 beats per minute on average at rest) in the late-3rd trimester. A full 15% of maternal cardiac output goes to the uterus at term. Maternal minute ventilation remains elevated at about 10.5 L per minute. Renal plasma flow declines bit in the 3rd trimester, but the GFR remains elevated.

Common obstetric complications and their management

Pregnancy loss—miscarriage, foetal death, and stillbirth

Case 1: Patient with intrauterine death at 22 weeks

A 24-year-old primigravida with systemic lupus erythematosus (SLE) and a history of deep venous thrombosis presents with a foetal death at 22 weeks of gestation. Ultrasound examination shows that the foetus is small-for-gestational-age and that oligohydramnios is present. The pregnancy was conceived during a period of SLE remission. The patient's antiphospholipid antibody status had not been previously investigated.

Case discussion

Pregnancy loss is a common reproductive outcome in humans—at least 30% of spontaneously conceived pregnancies fail. Most pregnancy losses occur before the missed menses that typically heralds the patient's recognition of pregnancy, but 10–15% of conceptions are lost after recognition of pregnancy, usually within the first 12 weeks of gestation. Among these, most fail as a result of failure of the embryo to develop or death of the embryo prior to 10 weeks of gestation, though the clinical features of pregnancy loss may not ensue for up to several weeks. Traditionally, the term miscarriage has been used to describe pregnancy loss prior to 20 weeks of gestation. More recently, we and others have used the term miscarriage to specifically indicate the loss of the conceptus prior to 10 weeks of gestation. The intrauterine death of a conceptus that has grown to 10 weeks of gestation or beyond is a foetal death, an event that complicates approximately 2% of all pregnancies. The delivery of a dead foetus at or beyond 20 weeks traditionally has been referred to as 'stillbirth'. Overall, most foetal deaths occur between the 10th and 15th week. From 16 weeks forward, approximately 1% of live foetuses expire in utero. After 20 weeks, foetal deaths occur in approximately 5–7 per 1,000 births in the general US population.

Within the general obstetric population, variables well recognized to influence pregnancy loss include maternal age and prior pregnancy loss. Pregnancy loss rates increase with increasing maternal age. Even among women with no prior pregnancy losses, the likelihood of miscarriage per pregnancy exceeds 20% by age 36 years and approaches 40% by age 40 years. At least half of miscarriages in the general obstetric population are chromosomally abnormal (aneuploid), and embryonic developmental and sub-chromosomal abnormalities are frequently found in miscarriage tissue with normal karyotypes.

Pregnancy loss prior to 10 weeks of gestation, i.e. miscarriage, is not a prominent feature of SLE or rheumatoid arthritis (RA), though disease activity in early pregnancy may predispose to miscarriage in a given pregnancy. Recurrent miscarriage is a clinical feature of APS, and some, but not all, studies suggest that maternal treatment with a heparin agent and low-dose aspirin (LDA) decreases the likelihood of miscarriage when prescribed early in gestation.

Foetal death rates are increased in relation to advancing maternal age and prior foetal death, as well as with obesity, smoking, chronic hypertension, insulin-requiring diabetes, and black race. For example, stillbirths are twice as likely in women more than 35–39 years of age compared to those less than 35 years of age and 1.5–3 times as likely in women with a prior stillbirth. Foetal death may be due to foetal infections, chromosomal abnormalities, syndromes of a Mendelian or polygenic origin, uterine malformations (e.g. uterine septum), or foeto-maternal haemorrhage.

Foetal death is also more likely in women with SLE and in women with primary APS. Lupus anticoagulant (LA) or positive tests for LA as well as anticardiolipin and anti-beta2-glycoprotein I are strong predictors of a risk for foetal death. Other risk factors include active lupus during pregnancy, maternal hypertension, and gestational hypertensive disease. The latter is more likely to occur in women with a history of lupus nephritis. Foetal death associated with APS is typically associated with foetal growth restriction and oligohydramnios, features of placental insufficiency, as well as severe gestational hypertension conditions.

Foetal death also may occur as a result of cardiac failure in pregnancies complicated by congenital complete heart block (CCHB). In such cases, the foetus demonstrates not only complete heart block, but also diminished ventricular function secondary to endomyocardial fibroelastosis. Foetal death in this setting is characterized by the presence of hydrops foetalis, i.e. progressively worsening oedema in soft tissues and serous cavity effusions.

Placental insufficiency and foetal growth restriction

Case 2: Patient with previous lupus nephritis and placental insufficiency

A 31-year-old woman is in her third pregnancy at 32 weeks of gestation. She has a history of lupus nephritis and has been on antihypertensive medication for over a decade. She is antiphospholipid antibody negative. During the pregnancy, she was maintained on labetalol, 200 mg three times daily. Her home blood pressures have been in 135/85 mm Hg range on average, and more recently have been 140–90 mm Hg. Obstetric ultrasound assessment finds the foetus to have an estimated foetal weight falling at the 5th percentile for 32 weeks of gestation and the 4-quadrant amniotic fluid volume index is 4 cm (indicative of oligohydramnios). Foetal umbilical artery Doppler waveform analysis finds absence of diastolic blood flow.

Case discussion

The maternal-placental circulation bathes the foetal villi with maternal blood so as to provide nutrients and gas exchange for the developing foetus. The placenta actively transports glucose, amino acids, and free fatty acids from the maternal to the foetal circulation. The rate of foetal growth accelerates at 24–28 weeks and slows somewhat after 32 weeks of gestation. Most foetal fat gain, however, occurs after 28 weeks of gestation.

Poor placental vascularization in the 1st and 2nd trimester may manifest itself as foetal growth restriction as the pregnancy advances and as the foetal growth demands increase. This condition is known as 'uteroplacental insufficiency' or, more simply, 'placental insufficiency'. Placental insufficiency is the single most common cause of foetal growth restriction in developed countries. Foetal growth restriction secondary to placental insufficiency typically involves asymmetric growth restriction—restricted somatic growth with sparing of foetal head growth. Such foetuses have smaller abdominal circumference measurements with relatively normal head measurements.

Though the mechanisms of poor placental vascularization are incompletely understood, placental insufficiency is well known to be associated with maternal hypertensive or vascular conditions, including maternal renal disease of diverse aetiologies ranging from acquired nephritis to inherited nephropathies. APS is associated with placental insufficiency and its manifestation. Indeed, early delivery for placental insufficiency is one clinical criterion for APS. Animal models of APS indicate that the poor placentation seen in this condition is associated with inflammation at the maternal-foetal interface, with activation of the complement system.

Other aetiologies of restricted foetal growth include inherent conditions of the foetus, such as foetal chromosomal, or genetic conditions, and foetal infection. The pattern of foetal growth restriction in such cases is typically symmetric in nature—both somatic and head growth are decreased. Low pre-pregnancy maternal weight or poor weight gain in pregnancy also are associated with impaired foetal growth, as are maternal smoking, cocaine use, and heavy alcohol use.

Management varies depending upon the severity of the placental insufficiency and the gestational age at which it occurs. At early gestational ages, e.g. 26 weeks of gestation, expectant management with close foetal surveillance using serial non-stress tests or biophysical profile tests, as well as umbilical artery Doppler waveform analysis, is common practice, given that the risks of pre-term birth are clinically concerning. In the case presented previously, the patient's history of lupus nephritis and chronic hypertension are known to increase the risk of placental insufficiency. Likely management would include antenatal steroids to enhance foetal maturity followed by delivery approximately 48 hours later.

Hypertensive disorders of pregnancy—gestational hypertension and pre-eclampsia

Case 3: Patient with thrombotic APS and pre-eclampsia

A 27-year-old woman with APS is now 26 weeks of gestation in her first pregnancy. Her diagnosis of APS was made at the time of a spontaneous DVT 5 years ago when she was found to be repeatedly positive for LA, as well as moderate-to-high titres of immunoglobulin G (IgG) anticardiolipin and IgG anti-beta2-glycoprotein I antibodies. A haematologist has been treating her with long-term anticoagulation, and she was switched to full anticoagulation doses of a low-molecular-weight heparin in very early pregnancy. She is also taking LDA. The patient now presents to labour and delivery with an initial blood pressure of 163/102 mmHg. Her AST and ALT are 2-to-3-fold normal and her platelet count is $74,000 \times 10^9$/L. A spot urine protein–creatinine ratio is 1.7.

Case discussion

Hypertensive disorders complicate 2–8% of pregnancies in unselected obstetric patients and are a major cause of maternal and foeto-neonatal morbidity and mortality. The two most common forms of hypertensive disorders of pregnancy are gestational hypertension and pre-eclampsia, with the latter historically defined as gestational hypertension accompanied by proteinuria. More recently, the American College of Obstetricians and Gynecologists (ACOG) states that gestational hypertension associated with certain 'severe' features should be diagnosed as 'pre-eclampsia with severe features' even if proteinuria is not present (Box 6.1) (1). Hypertensive disorders of pregnancy are more common among women with SLE, APS, and those with a history of renal disease of virtually any aetiology, including autoimmune, as well as among women with chronic hypertension.

The gestational hypertensive disorders present as new elevation of maternal blood pressure to or more than a systolic of 140 mm Hg or a diastolic of 90 mm Hg after 20 weeks of gestation and present on two more occasions at least 4 hours apart (1). Gestational hypertension in women with chronic essential hypertension manifests by worsening hypertension and other clinical features in the second half of pregnancy. As previously noted, pre-eclampsia is distinguished from gestational hypertension by the presence of new proteinuria (300 mg/dL in a 24-hours collection or a protein–creatinine ratio of 0.30 or more) or by the occurrence of any of several other severe clinical features (Box 6.1) (1). One of the more severe forms of pre-eclampsia is the syndrome of haemolysis (usually marked by an elevated LDH >600 IU/L) elevated liver enzymes, and low platelet count, known as haemolysis, elevated liver enzymes, low platelets (HELLP) syndrome. Eclampsia is the convulsive manifestation of gestational hypertensive disease and presents as new onset tonic-clonic, focal, or multifocal seizures in the absence of other causes.

Box 6.1 Severe features of gestational hypertensive disease indicating a diagnosis of severe pre-eclampsia

- Systolic blood pressure of 160 mm Hg or more, or diastolic blood pressure of 110 mm Hg or more on two occasions at least 4 hours apart (unless antihypertensive therapy is initiated before this time)
- Thrombocytopenia (platelet count less than $100,000 \times 10^9/L$)
- Impaired liver function as indicated by abnormally elevated blood concentrations of liver enzymes (to twice the upper limit normal concentration), and severe persistent right upper quadrant or epigastric pain unresponsive to medication and not accounted for by alternative diagnoses
- Renal insufficiency (serum creatinine concentration more than 1.1 mg/dL or a doubling of the serum creatinine concentration in the absence of other renal disease)
  - Pulmonary oedema
- New onset headache unresponsive to medication and not accounted for by alternative diagnoses
- Visual disturbances

Gestational hypertensive disorders may occur in a variety of seemingly unrelated clinical circumstances, including otherwise normal nulliparous women, pregnancies with multifoetal gestations, women with chronic renal disease, women with obesity, women with APS, and others. The pathophysiology of hypertensive disease remains unclear, though experts hold that a key event is abnormal placental vascularization leading to abnormal maternal-placental circulation. In this regard, the pathophysiology overlaps with that of placental insufficiency leading to foetal growth restriction, and the two conditions frequently coexist. One plausible theory is that the foeto-placental response to inadequate maternal-placental circulation is the elaboration of vasoactive substances that promote increased blood flow to the placenta. Mechanisms leading to abnormal placental vascularization are likely varied but exaggerated inflammatory responses at the maternal-foetal interface may be particularly important to the predisposition to hypertensive disorders of pregnancy among certain autoimmune populations.

Appropriate management of gestational hypertensive disorders requires an understanding of risks, application of preventive measures, and identification of the onset and severity of the condition. Among women with autoimmune disorders, common risk factors for gestational hypertension and pre-eclampsia are shown in Box 6.2. Some experts suggest using uterine artery Doppler indices and/or maternal circulating angiogenic factors to predict pre-eclampsia, but proof of improved outcomes is lacking. Preventive measures are limited, though the ACOG recommends LDA (1), 75–150 mg/day, beginning before 16 weeks of gestation and continuing until delivery in at-risk women without a contraindication to aspirin—this would include a majority of women with pre-existing autoimmune disease. It is worth noting that the treatment of gestational hypertension and pre-eclampsia with anti-hypertensives is not proven to influence disease progression or alter the timing of delivery.

Monitoring of maternal blood pressures and for signs and symptoms of gestational hypertensive disease is a cornerstone of appropriate management in women with autoimmune disorders. Maternal blood pressure determinations after 18–20 weeks of gestation at home is reasonable and common practice, and, of course, blood pressure determinations at prenatal visits is standard practice among women at risk. Once present, ongoing care of gestational hypertension and pre-eclampsia depends upon: 1) the gestational age, and 2) the severity of maternal disease or foetal consequences. For

---

Box 6.2 Some risk factors for gestational hypertensive disease in women with autoimmune conditions

- Antiphospholipid syndrome
- Systemic lupus erythematosus, especially with a history of renal involvement or current lupus flare
- Active nephritis
- Renal insufficiency
- Hypertension, especially that requiring treatment
- Thrombocytopenia

practical purposes, pregnancies that have reached 36–37 weeks are candidates for delivery, even in settings of mild foetal growth restriction or gestational hypertension. For gestational ages less than 36 weeks, delivery decisions are influenced by the severity of disease as manifest by such parameters as the degree of blood pressure (BP) elevation or the presence of severe features. When expectant management is deemed appropriate, close foetal surveillance using serial non-stress tests or biophysical profile tests is common practice, given that the risks of pre-term birth are clinically concerning. Antenatal steroid preparation of the foetus for delivery should be strongly considered. Medications such as hydralazine, labetalol, and nifedipine are used to control severely elevated maternal blood pressures. With infrequent exceptions at very early gestational ages, pre-eclampsia with severe features is an indication for delivery. Abnormal foetal testing results suggestive of foetal hypoxaemia are also an indication for delivery.

Though infrequent, one unique challenge of pregnancy management in women with SLE is distinguishing a lupus renal flare from pre-eclampsia. Laboratory and clinical evidence suggesting active renal disease support a diagnosis of a lupus flare, e.g. hypocomplementaemia or an active urine sediment. Proteinuria without an active sediment, new onset seizures, and features of HELLP syndrome suggest pre-eclampsia. Renal biopsy may aid in management and treatment decisions. Differentiation between lupus flare and pre-eclampsia/eclampsia (when possible) is important because treatments vary: pre-eclampsia with severe features is managed with delivery, whereas lupus flare is managed with medication.

In the case presented, the patient's history of APS and the presence of 'triple positive' aPL are predictive of pre-eclampsia with severe features in spite of her being treated with a heparin agent and LDA. The patient has clinical features of HELLP syndrome. Management would include treatment of maternal blood pressure, intravenous magnesium sulfate for seizure prophylaxis, administration of antenatal steroids to enhance foetal maturity, and delivery approximately 48 hours later.

Gestational diabetes

Gestational diabetes (GDM), carbohydrate intolerance that develops during pregnancy (2), is one of the most common complications of pregnancy in the US and is more likely to occur in women taking glucocorticoids. Other risks factors for GDM are shown in Box 6.3. Women with GDM are more likely to develop hypertensive disorders during pregnancy, undergo Caesarean delivery, and have a several-fold

---

Box 6.3 Risk factors for gestational diabetes

Body mass index >25, or >23 in Asian Americans
First-degree relatives with type 2 diabetes
High-risk race, e.g. African American, Latino, Native American, Pacific Islander
History of previous infant weighing 4 kg or more
History of gestational diabetes in prior pregnancy

higher risk of developing type 2 diabetes later in life. Offspring of women with GDM are more likely to be macrosomic (>4000 g birthweight), have obstetrical complications, develop hyperbilirubinaemia, and have increased risk for type 2 diabetes and metabolic syndrome later in life. Appropriate management of GDM reduces the obstetrical risks for both mother and baby.

Most experts recommend universal screening of pregnant women for GDM, though different screening approaches are offered in different countries. In the US, a two-step screening process is most commonly used (2). Women who do not have high-risk factors for GDM are routinely screened between 24 and 28 weeks of gestation using a 50 gram 1-hour oral glucose challenge. This test may be performed without regard to prandial state. Using a threshold of 135 or 140 mg/dL, those women who test positive subsequently undergo a 100 g, 3-hour oral glucose tolerance test in the fasting state. If any 2 of the 4 results are above diagnostic thresholds, a diagnosis of GDM is made. In some other countries, a one-step 75 g, 2-hour oral glucose tolerance test is employed.

Women at high risk for GDM, including women on glucocorticoids, should be screened in early pregnancy, and it is common practice to do this in the 1st trimester or early 2nd trimester. Options include the screening tests previously described, as well as the use of haemoglobin A1c. If the initial screening is negative, repeat screening should be done at 24–28 weeks.

Management of GDM is very similar to management of type 2 diabetes and begins with dietary modification, enhanced activity, and glucose monitoring. Insulin is the preferred pharmacological treatment recommended by ACOG inasmuch as it is time-tested and does not cross the placenta. Many practitioners in the US first try metformin in the management of mild GDM. Other oral agents are either not preferred or of unknown impact on the foetus. Treatment goals and related improvement in obstetric outcomes are provided in the Practice Bulletin from ACOG (2).

Pre-term birth

Pre-term birth (PTB), birth before 37 weeks of gestation, is the leading cause of perinatal and infant serious morbidity and mortality worldwide. Spontaneous PTB occurs as a consequence of the spontaneous onset of labour or pre-term premature rupture of membranes (PPROM) with subsequent labour, with some cases preceded by asymptomatic uterine bleeding or cervical shortening. The pathophysiology of spontaneous PTB is poorly understood and likely multifactorial in nature. In the US, the rate of PTB varies with the population being studied, but is approximately 10% overall. Indicated PTB is initiated by providers because of maternal or foetal concerns for which delivery is judged to be the best balance of risks and benefits, e.g. pre-eclampsia with severe features at 34 weeks of gestation.

Women with certain autoimmune conditions, particularly SLE, are at risk for both spontaneous and indicated PTB. Women with SLE face a 2–3-fold increased risk of PTB, with important variables including disease activity and history of lupus nephritis. Women with mild-to-moderate SLE in remission have a spontaneous PTB risk that is lower, quite similar to the risk in the general obstetric population. Women with APS have an elevated high rate of indicated PTB due to gestational hypertensive disease or placental insufficiency; those with LA or who are triple positive are at particularly higher risk.

Management of patients at risk for PTB requires close clinical assessment, adequate patient education, and thoughtful medical planning. Women at risk for spontaneous pre-term birth typically undergo cervical length measurements in the mid-trimester, with subsequent management steps base in part on whether or not the cervix is 'short'. Those at risk because of a previous spontaneous PTB of a singleton pregnancy are treated with weekly injections of 17-hydroxyprogesterone beginning at 16–24 weeks of gestation (3). Once a significant increased risk of PTB is found, considerations include the administration of antenatal steroids to enhance foetal maturity. Thus, a woman with either cervical shortening, symptoms of pre-term labour, or the onset of pre-eclampsia with severe features will be a candidate for antenatal steroids. Women with symptoms of pre-term labour are managed as inpatients and typically receive a course of magnesium sulfate infusion for neonatal neuroprophylaxis, as well as tocolytic agents such as nifedipine, though proof of efficacy is lacking for the latter. Women with PPROM are also managed as inpatients and are similarly treated with antenatal steroids and magnesium neuroprophylaxis, as well as an antibiotic regimen that may aid in delaying the onset of labour. The ultimate goals of management are: 1) to prepare the foetus for life as a pre-term neonate, and 2) safely delay delivery.

Selected special circumstances related to autoimmune disease in pregnancy

Case 4: Patient with anti-SSA antibodies

A 31-year-old woman with SLE not pregnant before is known to be positive for anti-SSA antibodies. Her SLE is mild-to-moderate in nature by history, she has no history of renal involvement, and she has been in remission for over 18 months. She understands that there is a risk of CCHB and would like you to formulate a strategy during her pregnancy for assessing and managing this concern.

Congenital complete heart block (CCHB)

Case discussion

The presence of anti-SS-A and/or anti-SS-B autoantibodies poses a risk for foeto-neonatal lupus, the most serious manifestation of which is CHB. Anti-SS-A and/or anti-SS-B antibodies are found in one-quarter to one-third of women with SLE and most patients with Sjögren syndrome (SS). Among women positive for anti-SS-A and/or anti-SS-B antibodies, but without a prior history of foeto-neonatal lupus, the risk of CHB is low, approximately 2%. However, among women who have previously had a pregnancy complicated by CHB, the risk for recurrent CHB is 15%–20%.

Most experts would recommend women with SLE or SS undergo assessment for anti-SS-A and/or anti-SS-B autoantibodies as a part of their pre-conceptional evaluation (those with a history of foeto-neonatal lupus will have already been evaluated). This can inform the patient and the provider in terms of risk. With regard to the development of foetal

CHB, possible preventive measures include: 1) administration of hydroxychloroquine (HCQ) to the mother (200–400 mg daily) from pre-conception or early pregnancy and continuing during pregnancy, and 2) serial assessment of the foetus for evolving cardiac conduction abnormalities. Retrospective evidence supports the premise that HCQ may reduce the risk of foetal-neonatal lupus, including CHB. A prospective treatment trial is near completion (NCT01379573). However, whether or not serial monitoring of the foetal PR interval via foetal echocardiographic assessment is clinically utilitarian remains a subject of controversy. Some experts believe that identification of 1st or 2nd degree foetal heart block may allow opportunity to avoid CHB by administration to the mother of dexamethasone, a glucocorticoid that crosses the placenta.

For women such as case 4, i.e. the presence of anti-Ro/SSA and/or anti-La/SSB antibodies with *no* history of an infant with congenital heart block or neonatal lupus (risk of CCHB ~2%), the current reproductive health guidelines created by the American College of Rheumatology (4) conditionally recommend the following:

- Obtain serial foetal echocardiography starting at weeks 16–18 through week 26.
- Consider treating the mother with hydroxychloroquine during pregnancy.

For women with anti-Ro/SSA and/or anti-La/SSB antibodies who have previously had a foetus or neonate with autoantibody-mediated CHB or neonatal lupus (risk of CHB 13–18%), the same reproductive health guidelines conditionally recommend the following:

- Obtain foetal echocardiography every week starting between weeks 16–18 through week 26.
- Treat with hydroxychloroquine during pregnancy.

If, in either of the situations outlined previously, the foetal echocardiogram is abnormal, the current guidelines suggest:

- If 1st degree heart block, treat with 4 mg of oral dexamethasone daily.
- If 2nd degree heart block, treat with 4 mg of oral dexamethasone daily.
- If isolated 3rd degree (complete) heart block (without other cardiac inflammation), do not treat with dexamethasone (for lack of any evidence of benefit with regard to the CHB).

It is worth emphasizing that not all experts agree with the previously mentioned monitoring and management scheme (5). Serial foetal echocardiography is costly and the benefits of treatment in preventing progression to 3rd degree heart block are, at best, uncertain. Moreover, multiple courses of fluorinated glucocorticoids may result in reduced body weight and size and a smaller head circumference (6).

Suspected APS

Case 5: Patient with antiphospholipid antibodies without clinical manifestations

A 37-year-old woman with a history of one prior miscarriage <10 weeks of gestation has seen an infertility specialist in order to achieve her pregnancy via in vitro fertilization and embryo transfer. She now has a positive pregnancy test and is 4–5 weeks of gestation. As a part of her evaluation, the infertility specialist determined that the patient had an IgM anticardiolipin result in the moderate positive range when she was tested 6 weeks ago. At that time, she was negative for LA, IgG anticardiolipin, and IgG anti-beta2-glycoprotein I antibodies. She is currently on a thromboprophylactic dose of a low molecular weight heparin and adamantly insists that this treatment is necessary for best foetal outcome.

Case discussion

The management of previously diagnosed, definite APS in pregnancy is discussed elsewhere in this text. In the case presented previously, the patient does not meet clinical criteria for APS, and, moreover, she has but a single positive antiphospholipid laboratory result. There exists no credible evidence that the patient should be treated with low-molecular-weight heparin for the purpose of either: 1) reducing her risk of possible aPL-mediated thrombosis, or 2) improving foetal outcome. At the same time, experts are not infrequently faced with the dilemma posed by the case presented: the patient being very concerned that a treatment is 'necessary'. Often, continuing the low-molecular-weight heparin is deemed reasonable based on patient insistence and the fact that adverse effects of this agent used in prophylactic doses are very infrequent. That said, continuing the low-molecular-weight heparin is non-evidence-based and fairly costly to the health care system at approximately $75 per day in the US, or about $15,000 to $20,000 per pregnancy so treated. Given the situation, one reasonable approach used in our clinics is to continue the low-molecular-weight heparin in the short term, repeat the anticardiolipin test at 12 weeks from the initial test (to confirm or refute a repeatedly positive result), and urge the patient to discontinue the heparin agent if the repeat test is negative, indeterminate, or low positive. Even if the repeat test is moderate positive, the patient does not meet criteria for APS, and strong consideration of discontinuing the heparin agent after a normal mid-trimester obstetric ultrasound is medically logical based on existing evidence.

Key messages

- An understanding of normal embryo-foetal development and maternal physiology of pregnancy aids in the management of pregnancy in women with rheumatic diseases.
- Women with SLE and/or APS are at risk for adverse pregnancy outcomes, including foetal death, gestational hypertensive disease, and placental insufficiency.
- Women with repeatedly positive tests for LA or who are triple positive for LA as well as medium-to-high titre anticardiolipin and anti-beta2-glycoprotein I antibodies are at increased risk for adverse pregnancy outcomes in spite of treatment with a heparin agent and LDA.
- Most experts recommend treating women with anti-Ro/SSA and/or anti-La/SSB antibodies with hydroxychloroquine during pregnancy as a preventive measure with regard to congenital heart block.
- In the absence of LA, the implications of low titre positive tests for anticardiolipin and anti-beta2-glycoprotein antibodies are uncertain.

Further reading

1. Gestational hypertension and preeclampsia. ACOG Practice Bulletin No. 202. American College of Obstetricians and Gynecologists. *Obstet Gynecol.* 2019;133:e1–25.
2. Gestational diabetes mellitus. ACOG Practice Bulletin No. 190. American College of Obstetricians and Gynecologists. *Obstet Gynecol.* 2018;131:e49–64.
3. Prediction and prevention of preterm birth. Practice Bulletin No. 130. American College of Obstetricians and Gynecologists. *Obstet Gynecol.* 2012;120:964–73.
4. Sammaritano LR, Bermas BL, Chakravarty EE, Chambers C, Clowse MEB, Lockshin MD, Marder W, et al. 2020 American College of Rheumatology Guideline for the Management of Reproductive Health in Rheumatic and Musculoskeletal Diseases. *Arthritis Rheumatol.* 2020;72:529–56.
5. Andreoli L, Bertsias GK, Agmon-Levin N, Brown S, Cervera R, Costedoat-Chalumeau N, Doria A, Fischer-Betz R, Forger F, Moraes-Fontes MF, Khamashta M, King J, Lojacono A, Marchiori F, Meroni PL, Mosca M, Motta M, Ostensen M, Pamfil C, Raio L, Schneider M, Svenungsson E, Tektonidou M, Yavuz S, Boumpas D, Tincani A. EULAR recommendations for women's health and the management of family planning, assisted reproduction, pregnancy and menopause in patients with systemic lupus erythematosus and/or antiphospholipid syndrome. *Ann Rheum Dis.* 2017 Mar;76(3):476–85.
6. Antenatal corticosteroid therapy for fetal maturation. Committee Opinion No. 713. American College of Obstetricians and Gynecologists. *Obstet Gynecol.* 2017;130:e102–109.

SECTION VII
VACCINATION BEFORE OR DURING PREGNANCY

7
Vaccination before or during pregnancy

Cara D. Varley and Kevin L. Winthrop

Introduction

This chapter focuses on the current recommendations, immunogenicity, and contra-indications for vaccination of women of childbearing age with rheumatic diseases who may be taking or considering initiation of disease-modifying antirheumatic drugs (DMARDs). Given the paucity of vaccine data in the pregnant population, some of the studies discussed include both men and women, children, and adults over 65 years old, which may not be generalizable to pregnant women.

Pre-conception

General

Given the many contraindications for various vaccines in pregnancy, all patients with rheumatological conditions who are of childbearing age should have their vaccine history reviewed prior to pregnancy if possible. Attempts should be made to ensure that they are up to date on childhood vaccines and vaccines recommended for rheumato-logical conditions prior to pregnancy and prior to the initiation of immunosuppressive therapy. Once pregnant or on certain immunosuppressive therapies (e.g. biologics), live vaccinations are generally contraindicated, and vaccines in general might have diminished immunogenicity. There is limited data on both the immunogenicity and safety of many vaccines in both pregnancy and during immunosuppressive therapy (see Table 7.1) (1–3).

Biological therapy

Hepatitis B virus (HBV) immune status is especially important to know in patients considering biological therapy as risk of reactivation is increased (1). All patients should be screened for HBV prior to starting immunosuppressive therapy. Those who lack prior exposure (negative HBV core antibody) and lack immunity (negative surface antibody) should be considered for HBV vaccination should risk factors for HBV be present (4).

There is limited clinical data evaluating the immunogenicity of vaccines in the setting of biological therapy, although some therapies have been shown to reduce responses to influenza, pneumococcal, or other vaccines. The influence of various biologics on these vaccines has recently been summarized (see Table 7.1).

Table 7.1 General vaccine recommendations and precautions for adults

Vaccine	DMARDs associated with decreased immunogenicity	Contraindications/precautions	Recommendations	Comments
Influenza, intramuscular attenuated vaccine	• rituximab (severe reduction) • abatacept • methotrexate (Friedman and Winthrop)	• None	• Yearly • High dose age >65 years (Moniz and Beigi; Kim and Hunter 2019)	Improved immunogenicity if methotrexate held for 2 weeks after vaccination (Park, Lee et al. 2018)
Pneumococcus				
pneumococcal conjugate vaccine (PCV13)	Decreased with adequate antibody levels in small (22 person) study of patients taking etanercept and methotrexate (Friedman and Winthrop)	• None	• One-time dose • Give ≥1 year after PPSV23 if given first (Kim and Hunter 2019)	Should be given before PPSV23 in vaccine naïve (Friedman and Winthrop)
pneumococcal polysaccharide vaccine (PPSV23)	• rituximab (severe reduction) • tofacitinib • methotrexate • >20 mg/d of prednisone (Friedman and Winthrop)	• None	• One-time dose ≥ 8 weeks to one year after PCV13 • Booster 5 years after 1st dose (Kim and Hunter 2019)	
Varicella Zoster Virus				
Varicella[v]	Limited data, however few reports in setting of juvenile rheumatoid arthritis (JRA) suggest decreased with: • methotrexate • prednisone • anti-tumour necrosis factor (TNF) therapy (Frenck and Seward)	• Pregnancy • Immunosuppressive therapy (Advisory Committee on Immunization Practices 2019)	• All nonimmune, unvaccinated patients (Kim and Hunter 2019)	Should not use acyclovir, famciclovir or valacyclovir 24 hours before and 14 days after vaccination (Advisory Committee on Immunization Practices 2019)

Hepatitis A virus (HAV)	Limited data suggests decreased with: • anti-TNF therapy • methotrexate (Askling, Rombo et al.)	• None	Anyone at risk for HAV or desires immunity, including: • homelessness • chronic liver disease • clotting factor disorders • travel to endemic areas • close contact with an international adoptee in the first 60 days after arrival from an endemic country • injection or non-injection drug use • work with HAV in a laboratory or with animals infected with HAV (Kim and Hunter 2019)	Screen for HAV IgG, if negative then vaccinate
Hepatitis B virus (HBV)	• anti-TNF therapy (Friedman and Winthrop)	• Heplisav-B during pregnancy given lack of available data (Kim and Hunter 2019)	Anyone at risk for HBV or desires immunity, including: • sexual partner with HBV • household contact with HBV • >1 sexual partner in the past 6 months • treatment of a sexually transmitted disease • intravenous drug use • health care worker • travel to endemic areas • diabetes	Screen for HBV sAb, sAg, cAb[≠] if negative then consider vaccination (Friedman and Winthrop)

(continued)

Table 7.1 Continued

Vaccine	DMARDs associated with decreased immunogenicity	Contraindications/ precautions	Recommendations	Comments
			• HIV • end stage renal disease • chronic liver disease (Schillie, Vellozzi et al. 2018; Kim and Hunter 2019)	
Human papillomavirus (HPV)	Seroconversion of 100% in small cohort of mild to moderate SLE patients taking: • prednisone 15 mg/day • hydroxychloroquine 400 mg/day. (Dhar, Essenmacher et al.)	• Pregnancy • None for immunosuppression (Friedman and Winthrop; Kim and Hunter 2019)	• Female age 11–26 years (Friedman and Winthrop; Kim and Hunter 2019)	
Tetanus toxoid, reduced diphtheria toxoid, and acellular pertussis (Tdap)	Limited data: lower antibody titres observed with: • azathioprine • mercaptopurine • anti-TNF therapy • baricitinib (tetanus) (Caldera, Saha et al.)	• None	• 27–36 weeks of gestation (Moniz and Beigi)	

* Severe allergic reaction (e.g. anaphylaxis) after a previous dose is a contraindication for all vaccines.

+ Moderate or severe acute illness with or without fever is a precaution for all vaccines.

¥ live attenuated vaccine.

*sAb = HBV surface antibody; sAg = HBV surface antigen; cAb = HBV core antibody.

Contraindications

Live attenuated vaccines are contraindicated in the setting of biological or immuno-suppressive therapy and should be administered 2–4 weeks before initiating therapy. There are case reports of incidental vaccination of patients on biological therapy with no adverse effects (varicella, live attenuated zoster vaccine, yellow fever), however the data is too sparse to fully assess the safety of routine vaccination (1, 3, 5, 6).

Pregnancy

General

Vaccines recommended during pregnancy include tetanus toxoid, reduced diphtheria toxoid, acellular pertussis (Tdap), and influenza. Tdap should be administered at 27–36 weeks of gestation in all pregnant women, primarily to protect the neonate with passive immunity. Seasonal influenza vaccine should be administered to all pregnant women, when seasonally available (7).

Biological therapy

There are currently no contraindications for Tdap or seasonal influenza vaccine in the setting of biological therapy.

Contraindications

Live attenuated vaccines are contraindicated in pregnancy due to concern for increased risks to the foetus and include the following: (3)

- measles, mumps, rubella (MMR)
- varicella-zoster (LAVZ)
- typhoid
- yellow fever.

Currently the human papillomavirus (HPV) vaccine is contraindicated due to lack of safety data in the setting of pregnancy (3).

Postpartum

General

If the patient did not receive Tdap during pregnancy, they should receive vaccination as soon as possible in the postpartum period (7).

Any live attenuated vaccines indicated prior to pregnancy should be administered postpartum, including MMR and varicella. Breastfeeding is not a contraindication to live attenuated vaccine administration (3).

It is also safe to complete or initiate the HPV vaccine series during the postpartum period if indicated for the patient (3).

Biological therapy, contraindications

Please refer to pre-conception biologics and contraindications section.

Consult cases

Case 1: Patient with RA who develops *Legionella* pneumonia at 18 weeks

A 26-year-old patient with rheumatoid arthritis (RA) and interstitial lung disease (ILD) maintained on prednisone 15 mg/day and azathioprine 100 mg/day develops *Legionella* pneumonia whilst in the 18th week of her second pregnancy. She recovers after completing 3 weeks of appropriate antimicrobial treatment.

Infectious disease consult questions

1. This patient never received any influenza nor pneumococcal vaccine. When is the best time to administer these immunizations following her recent bout of *Legionella* pneumonia?

This patient can currently receive both influenza and pneumococcal vaccination. 'Moderate or severe acute illness with or without fever' is currently a precaution and not a contraindication. If the patient's symptoms have resolved, it is appropriate to offer both vaccinations. For pneumococcus prevention, she should receive the PCV13 vaccine first followed by PPSV23 8 weeks to 12 months later (3). A randomized, double blind study did demonstrate lower immunoglobulins to PCV13 administered at the same time as influenza vaccination compared to PCV13 alone, however this study was done in patients over 65 years and the group receiving both vaccines concomitantly still achieved adequate immunogenicity. Accordingly, it is acceptable to administer both vaccines on the same visit (8).

2. The patient actively works as a farm help. Please comment on tetanus prophylaxis.

If the patient has an unknown date of last tetanus vaccine and has a potential risk of tetanus exposure, the Tdap vaccine can be administered now. She should not receive another dose of Tdap between 27–36 weeks. Tdap should only be administered once per pregnancy (7). In addition, if there is an ongoing outbreak of pertussis or a woman has an exposure to tetanus during pregnancy (e.g. steps on a rusty nail), the Tdap vaccine should be given at that time, even if prior to 27 weeks' gestation.

Case 2: Patient with lupus nephritis seeking vaccination travel advice

A 30-year-old reporter with stable lupus nephritis in the 1st trimester of pregnancy maintained on prednisone 15 mg/day and azathioprine 100 mg/day is travelling to parts of Southeast (SE) Asia on an assignment.

Infectious disease consult questions

1. What immunizations should and can she receive at this time?

Vaccine recommendations depend on duration of the trip and planned activities—animal exposures, rural vs urban areas, time of year, and specific countries. Many of the recommended vaccines for travel to rural areas of SE Asia are contraindicated or have precautions with pregnancy or immunosuppression given lack of clinical data. In this setting, referral to an outpatient infectious diseases provider as soon as travel plans are known is appropriate.

This patient should receive HBV and HAV vaccines, in addition to recommended vaccines based on Table 7.1. The inactivated typhoid vaccine should be considered, however, there is no information on the safety of this vaccine in pregnancy. The oral live attenuated typhoid vaccine is contraindicated in pregnancy and immunosuppression. Yellow fever vaccine is contraindicated in both pregnancy and immunosuppression (1, 5). Japanese encephalitis and rabies vaccines may be indicated based on anticipated activities, however pregnancy and immunosuppression are both precautions, and risk of infection vs risk of immunization needs to be discussed with the patient (5). In addition to vaccines, malaria prophylaxis may be needed, and the Centers for Disease Control and Prevention (CDC) currently has a warning for Zika virus in SE Asia (5).

Case 3: Patient with ITP with active hepatitis C infection

During her 1st trimester of an unplanned pregnancy, a 19-year-old with idiopathic thrombocytopenic purpura (ITP) on prednisone 30 mg/day develops active hepatitis C infection. Hepatitis A and B serology are all negative.

Infectious disease consult questions

1. What hepatitis immunization is recommended, if any? When can these be administered?
   - HBV and HAV vaccine series should be started now.
   - HBV surface antibody (≥10 mIU/mL) 1–2 months after completing the vaccine series to confirm immunity (4).

If failure to reach seroprotection, i.e. HBV surface antibody (≥10 mIU/mL) 1–2 months after completing the vaccine series, vaccination series should be repeated with repeat serological testing (4).

Case 4: Patient with SLE treated with rituximab seeking vaccination advice

A 34-year-old woman with known SLE diagnosed at the age of 28 with severe pancytopenia. At diagnosis, she was managed with intravenous methylprednisolone and plasma exchange and was stable on mycophenolate mofetil (MMF) 1 g daily for some years. Due to her wish to have a baby, the patient was switched to azathioprine. Unfortunately, the patient became thrombocytopenic (platelet nadir 20) and leukopenic. She was started on rituximab as she was reluctant to restart MMF.

Following her second dose of rituximab she achieved full B cell depletion and her platelet and leukocyte counts improved. Three months after her second dose of rituximab she finds out that she is 5 weeks pregnant. She has never received any hepatitis vaccinations, but would like to plan a trip to Asia to visit her family. Hepatitis A and B serologies were negative prior to initiating rituximab. She asks you if she can have HAV and HBV vaccination.

Infectious diseases consult questions

1. Can patient be given hepatitis A and B vaccination?
   - HBV and HAV vaccine series can be given, however there may be decreased immunogenicity in the setting of rituximab administration (currently no data available).
   - Giving vaccinations as far away as possible from the last rituximab dose will help maximize responses. Consider waiting at least 3 months from the last rituximab dose and ideally 2 weeks prior to the next rituximab dose if time allows.
   - HBV surface antibody (≥10 mIU/mL) 1–2 months after completing the vaccine series to confirm immunity (4).
   - In addition, given plans for travel, referral to an outpatient infectious diseases provider is appropriate to determine need for additional prophylaxis and provide infection prevention counselling.

If failure to reach seroprotection, i.e. HBV surface antibody (≥10 mIU/mL) 1–2 months after completing the vaccine series, vaccination series should be repeated with repeat serological testing (4).

Key messages

- Attempts should be made to administer recommended vaccines prior to pregnancy and initiation of immunosuppressive therapy.

- In general, live attenuated vaccines are contraindicated in pregnancy and with immunosuppression, especially biologics.
- There is limited safety and efficacy data for many inactivated, toxoid, and subunit/conjugate vaccines in the setting of pregnancy and biological therapy. Patients may not have an appropriate response and risks/benefits of receiving the vaccine must be weighed against risk of infection.
- Immunomodulating drugs, especially rituximab, can reduce vaccine immunogenicity, however there is limited or no clinical trial data on the effects of many available biological agents.
- Patients travelling out of the country with both immunosuppression and pregnancy should be referred to an infectious disease physician as soon as travel plans are known.

Further reading

1. Friedman MA, Winthrop KL. Vaccines and disease-modifying antirheumatic drugs: Practical implications for the rheumatologist. *Rheum Dis Clin N Am*. 2007;43(1):1–13.
2. Advisory Committee on Immunization Practices A. General Best Practice Guidelines for Immunization: Best Practices Guidance of the Advisory Committee on Immunization Practices (ACIP). *CDC*. 2019 (see https://www.cdc.gov/vaccines/acip/recommendations.html [updated 10 January 2019]).
3. Kim DK, Hunter P. Advisory Committee on Immunization Practices recommended immunization schedule for adults aged 19 years or older—United States, 2019. *MMWR Morb Mortal Wkly Rep*. 2019;68(5):115–18.
4. Schillie S, Vellozzi C, Reingold A, Harris A, Haber P, Ward JW, et al. Prevention of Hepatitis B virus infection in the United States: Recommendations of the Advisory Committee on Immunization Practices. *MMWR Recomm Rep*. 2018;67(1):1–31.
5. Centers for Disease Control and Prevention C. CDC Health Information for International Travel 2018. In: Brunette GW, ed. *CDC Yellow Book 2018*: Oxford: Oxford University Press, 2018.
6. Frenck RW, Jr., Seward JF. Varicella vaccine safety and immunogenicity in patients with juvenile rheumatic diseases receiving methotrexate and corticosteroids. *Arthritis Care Res (Hoboken)*. 2016;62(7):903–6.
7. Moniz MH, Beigi RH. Vaccination During Pregnancy. *Obstet Gynecol Surv*. 2016; 71(3):178–86.
8. Schwarz TF, Flamaing J, Rumke HC, Penzes J, Juergens C, Wenz A, et al. A randomized, double-blind trial to evaluate immunogenicity and safety of 13-valent pneumococcal conjugate vaccine given concomitantly with trivalent influenza vaccine in adults aged >65 years. *Vaccine*. 2014;29(32):5195–202.
9. Donegan K, King B, Bryan P. Safety of pertussis vaccination in pregnant women in UK: Observational study. *BMJ*. 2014;349:g4219.

SECTION VIII
RARE DISEASES IN PREGNANCY

8.1

Systemic lupus erythematosus

Karen Schreiber and Monika Østensen

Case 1: Systemic lupus erythematosus (SLE) quiescent disease prior to conception and hydroxychloroquine (HCQ) adherence

A 26-year-old nurse of Hispanic origin presents in your clinic. She has systemic lupus erythematosus (SLE) which was diagnosed at the age of 21 based on skin rashes, hair loss, mouth ulcers, and arthralgia. She was subsequently found to be antinuclear antibody (ANA) positive, and has a persistent mild leukopenia and thrombocytopenia. Her antiphospholipid antibodies (aPL) and extractable nuclear antigens (ENA) were previously negative. She has had a musculoskeletal flare of her SLE 4 months ago but has otherwise been stable. She experienced her flare whilst she was on a summer holiday and believes it was triggered by sun exposure.

She is keen to become pregnant, but is generally worried about having a baby, her medications and their compatibility with pregnancy. She asks you if she can stop her HCQ before pregnancy. She takes only over-the-counter vitamin tablets including folic acid.

Case discussion

This patient has SLE with musculoskeletal involvement, without any history of renal or lung involvement. She has had a minor flare 4 months ago, and would like to become pregnant, but is worried about her medications and whether these are compatible with pregnancy.

There are two important things to address in this case; firstly she requires careful counselling about her disease activity and its implications for pregnancy and secondly she requires reassurance about her medication.

SLE disease activity in women planning pregnancy

Pregnancy outcome in women with SLE has unquestionably improved with a significant decrease in pregnancy morbidity over the last five decades from 40% in the early 1960s to less than 15% in recent years (1). Pregnancy counselling, treatment during pregnancy, follow-up during pregnancy, and postpartum have inevitably contributed to the improved pregnancy outcomes.

Recent data from the Predictors of Pregnancy Outcome: Biomarkers in Anti-phospholipid Antibody Syndrome and Systemic Lupus Erythematosus (PROMISSE) study has given answers to some long-discussed questions. The PROMISSE cohort is so far the largest prospective multicentre cohort study of pregnant women with underlying stable SLE (2) and included 385 women with a diverse ethnic and socioeconomic background recruited from nine centres in total (eight centres across the United States and one in Canada) who were followed at monthly intervals during pregnancy. Outcome measures were adverse pregnancy outcomes defined as foetal or neonatal death, birth before 36 weeks due to placental insufficiency, hypertension, or pre-eclampsia; and small-for-gestational-age (SGA) neonate (birth weight <5th percentile). Disease activity was assessed with the Systemic Lupus Erythematosus Pregnancy Disease Activity Index (SLEPDAI) and the Physician's Global Assessment (PGA). The aim of the study was to identify risk factors for adverse pregnancy outcomes due to SLE or/and the presence of aPL. Patients included into the PROMISSE cohort had quiescent SLE (and patients with a urine protein–creatinine ratio >1000 mg/g, creatinine level greater than 1.2 mg/dL and prednisone use greater than 20 mg/day, and twin pregnancies were excluded from participation). The flare rate in the 2nd and 3rd trimesters of women participating in the study were 2.5% and 3% respectively, which is much lower than other studies previously have reported. This emphasizes two things: the recommendation of pre-pregnancy counselling and conceiving during a disease quiescent phase. In 81% of the study participants Buyon et al. found women to have a successful pregnancy outcome, in other words, the child was born alive delivered after 36 weeks of gestation and was in at least the 5th percentile for birth weight.

The PROMISSE study also highlights the remarkable difference in pregnancy outcomes across ethnic groups. Attributes of women with successful pregnancy outcomes were non-Hispanic white origin, a negative lupus anticoagulant, not treated for hypertension at study entry, no or low disease activity, and a platelet count of at least 100 10^9 cells/L. In comparison, women who were not of non-Hispanic white origin had more than double the risk of developing one or more adverse pregnancy outcomes; in women of African (N = 78) and Hispanic (N = 58) descent, poor foetal outcomes were found in 27.4% and 20.6%, respectively.

Other predictors of poor pregnancy performance were antihypertensive drug use at baseline, the presence of lupus anticoagulant, severe clinical flare of SLE during pregnancy, mild or moderate clinical flare, moderate clinical disease activity at baseline, and thrombocytopenia. Interestingly, commonly used serological variables to anticipate clinical outcomes, such as complement levels and anti-double-stranded DNA (dsDNA) positivity were not associated with adverse pregnancy outcomes. However, anti-ds-DNA was analysed as a dichotomized variable, whereas the clinical use mainly is based in the titre tendency. Complement levels in turn are difficult to interpret in pregnancy due to the influence of oestrogen in particular and, in the PROMISSE cohort, low complement levels at baseline were more often seen in patients with adverse pregnancy outcomes. In conclusion, this study provides reassurance for women with stable disease and their responsible clinicians that pregnancy outcomes are favourable.

The general advice is that women should be stable for at least 6 months prior to conception. SLE activity around conception or less than 6 months prior to conception is associated with an increased risk of SLE flare during pregnancy and 3 months postpartum (3).

In our previously mentioned case we should therefore advise our patient to postpone pregnancy until she has been stable for at least 6 months. Most experts would agree that patients who require switch of immunosuppression prior to pregnancy should be monitored for their response to the pregnancy-compatible choice of immunosuppression in order to ensure that the disease remains stable. In our case the patient remains on HCQ, which can be taken periconception, during pregnancy, and during lactation. She requires reassurance about the safety of the use of HCQ during pregnancy and should be informed that there is a considerable risk for SLE flare in case she discontinues the drug. For further information on the use of antirheumatics during pregnancy and lactation see Chapter 3.1.

Case 2: SLE and contraception

A 34-year-old teacher presents in your clinic. She has SLE and mixed connective tissue disease (MCTD) overlap which was diagnosed at the age of 24 based on Raynaud's, 'puffy hands', skin rashes, hair loss, mouth ulcers, and arthralgia. She is ANA, dsDNA, and U1-ribonucleoprotein (U1RNP) positive and is also known to have persistently positive lupus anticoagulant (without any clinical manifestation of antiphospholipid syndrome (APS)). She has had two successful pregnancies and asks for your advice regarding the oral contraceptive pill. She is a non-smoker, has a body mass index (BMI) of 25, no history of migraine, and no family history of thrombosis.

Case discussion

This patient would like your advice on the use of the oral contraceptive pill in relation to her SLE. She has persistent aPL, which should be taken into consideration when assessing which contraceptive method is most suitable in her situation. In most countries the available methods of contraception include long-acting reversible contraception, such as the implant or intrauterine device (IUD), hormonal contraception, such the pill (progesterone only or combined pill), or the Depo Provera injection, and barrier methods (such as condoms). There may, however, be local differences in availability and prices which may impact the local recommendations on contraception.

SLE activity and contraception

It is well-known that SLE has its preponderance for women of childbearing age (4); consequently, contraception and pregnancy is an important issue to address for the patient and the treating physician. According to the recent European League Against Rheumatism (EULAR) and American College of Rheumatology (ACR) guidelines, women with SLE and/or APS should be counselled about contraception, especially in view of preventing unplanned pregnancies whilst treated with potentially teratogenic medications and to prevent unwanted pregnancies during high disease activity periods. Effective contraceptive methods should therefore be discussed with the patient by weighing the individual risk factors, including general (hypertension, obesity, tobacco use, family history of hormonal-dependent cancers) and disease related risk factors, particularly disease activity and thrombotic risk (especially in women with aPL or APS) (5, 6).

SLE most commonly presents in women of childbearing age and, historically, one of the main concerns for women with SLE using hormonal contraceptives has been the concern that oestrogen containing medication may trigger SLE activity (7, 8).

Two randomized controlled trials (RCTs) have evaluated whether use of combined oral contraceptives (OCs) is associated with SLE disease activity. In a multicentre RCT, 183 women with SLE were randomized to either treatment with a 35 μg ethinyloestradiol triphasic combined oral contraceptive or an identical placebo (9). The 12-month severe flare rate was not different between the two groups nor were any other measures of disease severity over the 12-month period. None of these RCTs included women with active SLE; the results indicate that at least for women with stable SLE, the use of hormonal contraceptives, either combined oestrogen and progestogen or progestogen-only, does not trigger SLE flares.

In a second single-blind, non-placebo, RCT 54 women with SLE were randomized to the combined oral contraceptive pill (30 μg ethinylestradiol/150 μg levonorgestrel), 54 to progestogen-only pill (30 μg levonorgestrel), and 54 to the IUD (10). There was no difference in global disease activity at any of the follow-up points in any of the treatment arms over a period of 1 year and there was no difference in the likelihood of any SLE flare in the treatment arms.

In patients persistently positive for aPL or APS however, the use of oestrogen containing medications should be avoided for their increased risk of thrombosis. It is only in rare exceptional cases that oestrogen containing medications should be used in patients with thrombotic APS provided that these patients are adequately anticoagulated (such an example could be male to female gender modification which requires oestrogen treatment). There are no RCTs addressing this question in patients with aPL or APS only, but since any modifiable thrombotic risk factors should be avoided in these patients, most experts agree that oestrogen containing medications should be avoided (11). The best evidence assessing the risk of thrombosis in patients with aPL and SLE stems from case-control data including 157 patients, of which 131 were women, and in which the presence of lupus anticoagulant was amongst the strongest risk factors for the development of thrombosis, see (5, 11).

In our case the patient has quiescent disease, but is known to have persistent aPL. She should therefore be advised to avoid any oestrogen containing oral contraceptive and advised to either use barrier methods, the progesterone only pill, or IUD. It is also worth mentioning that women with aPL who experience post-menopausal symptoms should avoid oestrogen containing hormonal replacement therapy (HRT), and that post-menopausal symptoms therefore should be managed with alternative non-oestrogen containing medications.

Key messages

- Women with SLE who are planning to become pregnant should be in remission for at least 6 months prior to conception.
- Women with quiescent SLE prior to pregnancy often have successful pregnancies.
- Women with aPL and APS should avoid oestrogen containing medications (such as oestrogen containing oral contraceptive pill and HRT).

Further reading

1. Clark CA, Spitzer KA, Laskin CA. Decrease in pregnancy loss rates in patients with systemic lupus erythematosus over a 40-year period. *J Rheumatol*. 2005;32(9):1709–12.
2. Buyon JP, Kim MY, Guerra MM, et al. Predictors of pregnancy outcomes in patients with lupus: A cohort study. *Ann Intern Med*. 2015;163(3):153–63.
3. Kwok LW, Tam LS, Zhu T, Leung YY, Li E. Predictors of maternal and fetal outcomes in pregnancies of patients with systemic lupus erythematosus. *Lupus*. 2011;20(8):829–36.
4. Kaul A, Gordon C, Crow MK, et al. Systemic lupus erythematosus. *Nat Rev Dis Primers*. 2016;2:16039.
5. Andreoli L, Bertsias GK, Agmon-Levin N, et al. EULAR recommendations for women's health and the management of family planning, assisted reproduction, pregnancy and menopause in patients with systemic lupus erythematosus and/or antiphospholipid syndrome. *Ann Rheum Dis*. 2017;76(3):476–85.
6. Sammaritano LR, Bermas BL, Chakravarty EE, et al. American College of Rheumatology Guideline for the Management of Reproductive Health in Rheumatic and Musculoskeletal Diseases. *Arthritis Rheumatol*. 2020 Apr;72(4):529–556.
7. Rahman A, Isenberg DA. Systemic lupus erythematosus. *N Engl J Med*. 2008;358(9):929–39.
8. Wahren-Herlenius M, Dorner T. Immunopathogenic mechanisms of systemic autoimmune disease. *Lancet*. 2013;382(9894):819–31.
9. Petri M, Kim MY, Kalunian KC, et al. Combined oral contraceptives in women with systemic lupus erythematosus. *N Engl J Med*. 2005;353(24):2550–58.
10. Sanchez-Guerrero J, Uribe AG, Jimenez-Santana L, et al. A trial of contraceptive methods in women with systemic lupus erythematosus. *N Engl J Med*. 2005;353(24):2539–49.
11. Chopra N, Koren S, Greer WL, et al. Factor V Leiden, prothrombin gene mutation, and thrombosis risk in patients with antiphospholipid antibodies. *J Rheumatol*. 2002;29(8):1683–8.

8.2

Systemic lupus erythematosus and the risk of cardiovascular disease

Karen Schreiber and Søren Jacobsen

Case 1: Systemic lupus erythematosus (SLE) and the risk of future cardiovascular disease

A 29-year-old pharmacist presents in your pregnancy clinic. She was diagnosed with systemic lupus erythematosus (SLE) at the age of 16 based on musculoskeletal symptoms, including symmetrical small joint arthritis, photosensitivity, and a malar rash. There has never been renal involvement. Repeated tests for antiphospholipid antibodies (aPL) were negative. Her maintenance therapy includes hydroxychloroquine (HCQ) 200 mg daily, which she tolerates well. Two years previously she had a normal weight pre-term baby at week 29 due to pre-eclampsia, and she has since then had hypertension requiring antihypertensive therapy. She was regularly followed up due to her SLE and her known hypertension. Her routine urine tests were always negative for protein. Her mother had a myocardial infarction at the age of 49, however, she reported no other family members with cardiovascular disease (CVD). She has a body mass index (BMI) of 27 and smokes occasionally. Her lipid profile has in the past been within normal ranges. She is currently not planning for further pregnancies but is worried about her risk of CVD, as she has read some conflicting information on the internet. She asks you about your opinion on low-dose aspirin for the primary prevention of CVD.

Case discussion

This patient is worried about her possible risk for future CVD as she has SLE and a family history of a first-degree relative with premature CVD. The case of our patient directs attention towards three important subjects: firstly, it emphasizes the issue of risk of premature CVD in women with SLE, which is especially pronounced in women with aPL antibodies, a history of renal involvement and/or ischaemic placental dysfunction including pre-eclampsia, eclampsia, and intrauterine growth restriction (IUGR). Secondly, it highlights the important role of the physician to inform patients with SLE about this risk and the role of potentially modifiable cardiovascular risk factors in this particular situation. Thirdly, it shows the important role of patient education and patient empowerment in disease prevention. With regard to the latter, counselling about a future risk for any potential life-threatening disease requires careful and considerate counselling.

In general, women account for roughly 90% of patients with SLE and they are typically diagnosed when of childbearing age. Patients with SLE are at increased risk of premature CVD representing the major cause of morbidity and mortality in these patients (1, 2). Data suggest that cardiovascular events (CVEs) occur a decade earlier in women with SLE compared to women without SLE (2). Particularly, younger SLE patients with renal involvement are at increased risk with hazard ratios of about 45 which is 17 times higher than for those without renal involvement (3).

The occurrence of placenta-mediated complications has been described as the earliest clinically identifiable marker of a woman's increased risk of CVD in that the relationship of pre-eclampsia to the future development of CVD has been well established in the general population (4). Women with SLE have a higher risk for placenta-mediated adverse pregnancy outcomes, which includes gestational hypertension, pre-eclampsia, eclampsia, IUGR, and at worst intrauterine death. In more detail, the risk of pre-eclampsia in women with SLE is 3-fold higher compared to the general population and occurs in up to 20–30% of women with SLE. The risk for pre-eclampsia in women with SLE is associated to ethnicity (with women of Afro-Caribbean and Hispanic origin being at higher risk compared to Caucasian women), to the presence of pre-existing hypertension, renal involvement (in particular renal disease activity), and SLE disease activity in general. Population-based data from the Swedish Patient Registry indicate that women with SLE and a history of pre-eclampsia have a 2-fold greater risk of death from primary cardiovascular causes; this risk was over 3-fold when combined with pre-term delivery <34 weeks' gestation (5). A second study showed that pregnancy complicated by pre-eclampsia and pre-term delivery exerts an independent effect to increase the risk and accelerate the future development of CVEs in women with SLE (6).

There are currently two hypotheses associating placenta-mediated complications with the development of future CVD. One hypothesis is that pre-existing vascular dysfunction may predispose women to abnormal placentation in early pregnancy, which results in endothelial cell activation and subsequently results in hypoxia triggering the maternal generalized response syndrome seen as pre-eclampsia. A second hypothesis suggest that endothelial damage, caused by high levels of circulating anti-angiogenic factors and placentally derived microvesicles, directly leads to premature CVD. Circulating microvesicles have also been associated with the development of nephritis in SLE patients (7) providing clues for pre-eclampsia, lupus nephritis, and CVD sharing common pathogenic factors.

Pregnancy has therefore been suggested to play a pivotal role in the development of CVD: women who develop pre-eclampsia during pregnancy are four times more likely to develop hypertension later in life, and are twice as likely to develop heart disease, stroke, and thrombosis in the future compared to women with normal pregnancies (4).

Regarding our case, the patient actively seeks information regarding her risk, which indicates that she already is aware of a potential risk and possibly also is motivated for some lifestyle changes to minimize her future CVD risk. The usual modifiable CVD risk factors from the Framingham cohort are therefore a good starting point and you therefore advise her to continue her anti-hypertensive medication and to stop smoking. Further, you may suggest she be seen by a dietician to adjust her diet to achieve weight loss. Exercise is known to reduce blood pressure. However, there is a lack of data to suggest that the modification of these lifestyle factors is associated with a CVD risk reduction in women with SLE. Nevertheless, the European League Against Rheumatism (EULAR) recommends that the guidelines for the prevention of CVD for the general population are followed. The patient has no signs of active renal disease or aPL antibodies, which fortunately takes out these risk factors. However, the patient is also encouraged to continue adhering to her HCQ treatment; several observational studies indicate benefits of HCQ also in CVD risk protection. As to aspirin, recent data suggest that the role of low-dose aspirin in primary CVD prevention in the general population is not indicated and you therefore advise the patient against using it in the current situation.

Key messages

- Patients with SLE are at increased risk of premature CVD representing the major cause of morbidity and mortality in this patient group.
- Premature CVD is significantly pronounced in women with SLE who have a history of pre-eclampsia.
- The prevention of future CVD is particularly important in women with a previous pregnancy history complicated by pre-eclampsia.

Further reading

1. Urowitz MB, Bookman AA, Koehler BE, Gordon DA, Smythe HA, Ogryzlo MA. The bimodal mortality pattern of systemic lupus erythematosus. *Am J Med*. 1976;60(2):221–5.
2. Manzi S, Meilahn EN, Rairie JE, et al. Age-specific incidence rates of myocardial infarction and angina in women with systemic lupus erythematosus: Comparison with the Framingham Study. *Am J Epidemiol*. 1997;145(5):408–15.
3. Hermansen ML, Lindhardsen J, Torp-Pedersen C, Faurschou M, Jacobsen S. The risk of cardiovascular morbidity and cardiovascular mortality in systemic lupus erythematosus and lupus nephritis: A Danish nationwide population-based cohort study. *Rheumatology* (Oxford). 2017;56(5):709–15.
4. Bellamy L, Casas JP, Hingorani AD, Williams DJ. Pre-eclampsia and risk of cardiovascular disease and cancer in later life: Systematic review and meta-analysis. *BMJ*. 2007;335(7627):974.
5. Soh MC, Nelson-Piercy C, Dib F, Westgren M, McCowan L, Pasupathy D. Brief report: Association between pregnancy outcomes and death from cardiovascular causes in parous women with systemic lupus erythematosus: A study using Swedish population registries. *Arthritis Rheumatol*. 2015;67(9):2376–82.
6. Soh MC, Dib F, Nelson-Piercy C, Westgren M, McCowan L, Pasupathy D. Maternal-placental syndrome and future risk of accelerated cardiovascular events in Parous Swedish women with systemic lupus erythematosus—a population-based retrospective cohort study with time-to-event analysis. *Rheumatology* (Oxford). 2016;55(7):1235–42.
7. Rasmussen NS, Jacobsen S. Microparticles—culprits in the pathogenesis of systemic lupus erythematosus? *Expert Rev Clin Immunol*. 2018;14(6):443–5.

8.3

Antiphospholipid syndrome

Karen Schreiber and Savino Sciascia

Antiphospholipid syndrome (APS) is characterized by arterial and/or venous thromboses and/or obstetric morbidity in patients persistently positive for moderate to high titres of antiphospholipid antibodies (aPL) as outlined in the Sydney classification criteria (1). Patients with a history of obstetric morbidity are referred to as having 'obstetric APS' and those with any aPL-related thrombosis are referred to as 'thrombotic APS'. Those with positive antibodies but without any past obstetric or thrombotic events have not yet met any criteria, but may be at increased risk of developing thrombosis and/or adverse pregnancy events.

APS is considered as the major acquired thrombophilia which, unlike other thrombophilias, can affect the venous, arterial, or microvasculature. It is therefore not surprising that APS can present in various clinical ways. The most common venous thromboses include deep vein thrombosis (DVT) and pulmonary embolism (PE) whereas the most common arterial manifestations comprise stroke or transient ischaemic attacks (2). Thrombocytopenia and livedo reticularis are the most important haematological and dermatological presentations, respectively, and can be found in up to 20% of APS patients (2, 3).

Pregnancy morbidity includes unexplained recurrent (≥3 consecutive) 1st trimester pregnancy loss, any 2nd or 3rd trimester pregnancy loss, premature birth before 34 weeks of gestation due to conditions associated with ischaemic placental dysfunction such as severe pre-eclampsia, eclampsia, and foetal growth restriction. Pre-eclampsia, premature birth or foetal loss are the most common manifestations and are seen in 10–20% of APS pregnancies (2, 3).

The prevalence of aPL in normal healthy populations has been reported to range between 1–5%, whereas the prevalence of aPL has been reported as high as 30% in patients with other autoimmune conditions such as rheumatoid arthritis or systemic lupus erythematosus (SLE) (3).

The treatment of APS has long been subject of intense debate, due to fact that the understanding of the syndrome has increased over the years. In regard to the management of women with aPL planning pregnancy, the European League against Rheumatism (EULAR) published their recommendation in 2017 (4).

In the following section we will present three cases of women with different presentations of APS and discuss the current most common treatment practice and evidence.

Case 1: Recurrent early pregnancy loss

A 29-year-old nurse presents in your clinic. She has a history of four consecutive recurrent pregnancy losses before the 10th week of gestation. She has never taken any medications during any of these pregnancies. Moreover, she has persistent mild thrombocytopenia, and a test of aPL was positive for lupus anticoagulant and anticardiolipin IgG. She is very keen for a further pregnancy.

She has no other past medical history, is normal weight with a body mass index (BMI) of 23, and she has a healthy lifestyle. She takes only over-the-counter vitamin tablets including folic acid. On examination you note widespread livedo reticularis on her arms and thighs, which she has had for years. She denies sicca symptoms, joint pains, mouth ulcers, and fatigue, or any symptoms that would suggest any connective tissue disease.

You perform blood tests, and you confirm that she is positive for lupus anticoagulant and she has a high titre of anticardiolipin IgG antibodies. As her previous aPL test was performed over 12 weeks ago, you confirm that she is persistently aPL positive (as per current classification criteria). Her full blood count confirms a persistent mild thrombocytopenia.

Case discussion

This patient has experienced four recurrent consecutive early pregnancy losses and has not received any treatment during these pregnancies in the past. No other cause (such as genetic abnormality and infection) for her recurrent miscarriage has been found. She has persistent aPL and can therefore be classified as having obstetric APS. Her livedo reticularis is a common skin manifestation of APS.

The current recommendations for the treatment of women with persistent aPL and a history of recurrent consecutive 1st-trimester pregnancy loss (without previous thrombosis) include low-dose aspirin (LDA) (75–100 mg/day) +/- low-molecular-weight heparin (LMWH) (e.g. subcutaneous dalteparin, enoxaparin, nadroparin, or subcutaneous tinzaparin), or unfractionated heparin.

These recommendations are based on results from randomized, controlled trials of varying quality comparing LDA alone or in combination with heparin in women with aPL.

A summary of our treatment recommendations is outlined in Table 8.3.1.

The use of LDA +/- LMWH in pregnant women with aPL (with or without definite APS) have improved overall pregnancy outcome to live birth rates of >70%, but 20–30% of women with persistent aPL or APS develop pregnancy complications despite aspirin +/- heparin and therefore require careful multidisciplinary follow-up during pregnancy (EULAR).

Other medications to prevent pregnancy morbidity in women with persistent aPL (especially in women who develop further pregnancy morbidity despite treatment with aspirin and LMWH) include low-dose prednisolone, the antimalarial hydroxychloroquine (HCQ), or azathioprine (AZA). There is currently no international consensus about the order of choice of these agents. Retrospective clinical studies have reported a potential role for HCQ in pregnant women with APS, however, this observation needs confirmation from prospective randomized clinical trials. Intravenous immunoglobulin (IVIG) in the setting of obstetric APS has been studied in clinical trials, with no significant improvement in pregnancy outcomes and is therefore not recommended for use.

Table 8.3.1 Management of women with aPL and APS during pregnancy

Clinical manifestation	Treatment	Evidence
Persistent presence of aPL in women, first pregnancy or with previous normal pregnancies	Close monitoring of mother and foetus during pregnancy, with or without LDA	Decision on individual basis Data support the use of LDA to prevent PET in high-risk pregnancies
Persistent aPL positive and history of recurrent 1st trimester pregnancy loss (without previous thrombosis)	LDA with or without prophylactic heparin	Randomized controlled trials of varying quality
History of foetal loss or previous history of ischaemic placental mediated complications	LDA with prophylactic heparin	Randomized controlled trials of varying quality
Patients with thrombotic APS (venous or arterial)	LDA and intermediate or therapeutic dose LMWH	Based on one prospective observational study

aPL, antiphospholipid antibodies; APS, antiphospholipid syndrome; LDA, low-dose aspirin; LMWH, low-molecular-weight heparin; PTE, pre-eclampsia toxaemia.

All women with APS can potentially give birth naturally, unless there are obstetric reasons that suggest the opposite. Women with persistent aPL should receive thromboprophylaxis postpartum.

Subcutaneous LMWH is discontinued for most patients when spontaneous labour begins, or 12–24 hours before planned induction of labour or Caesarean delivery (12 hours for prophylactic dose; 24 hours for higher doses), consistent with an American College of Obstetricians and Gynecologists (ACOG) practice bulletin and an American Society of Hematology (ASH) guideline from 2018 (5, 6).

Case 2: Woman with a previous history of placental mediated complications

A 35-year-old pediatrician is referred to your clinic. She is worried and explains that she has a history of two early pregnancy losses before week 10 of gestation and has given birth to a severely growth-restricted baby girl at week 29 due to severe pre-eclampsia. She was subsequently diagnosed with APS based on her obstetric history and persistently positive tests for lupus anticoagulant over 12 weeks apart. She is very keen for a further pregnancy. She has no other past medical history, has a BMI of 20, and her blood pressure (BP) is normal.

You advise her to take aspirin and LMWH during her next pregnancy and you outline a close follow-up together with your obstetric colleagues. You also inform her that you will refer her for uterine artery Doppler ultrasound in the 2nd trimester. She has herself read some articles on the use of aspirin and heparin and would like to know your opinion on the available evidence.

Case discussion

Placental insufficiency is the failure of the placenta to deliver sufficient nutrients to the growing foetus and can manifest as intrauterine growth restriction (IUGR) and/or pre-eclampsia (PET) (see also Chapter 6). In the previously mentioned case the patient has a history of aPL-related placental insufficiency and PET. The current treatment recommendation for subsequent pregnancies would therefore be to treat her with LDA and LMWH (Table 8.3.1).

Most prospective observational cohort studies support the association of aPL with PET and placental insufficiency and data from a systematic meta-analysis showed that moderate to high levels of anticardiolipin (aCL) are associated with PET, and prospective and retrospective studies have shown that the persistent presence of high-titre aPL is associated with IUGR and pre-term deliveries. In turn, raised aPL was found in up to 50% of patients with a history of PET or IUGR (compared to 7% or less in healthy pregnant women).

The FRUIT-RCT is to date the only randomized controlled trial assessing the management and prevention of PET and intrauterine growth restriction in women with persistent aPL. The aim of the trial was to examine, if the combination of LMWH and aspirin reduces recurrent hypertensive disorders (HD) of pregnancy (including pre-eclampsia, eclampsia, or haemolysis, elevated liver enzymes, and a low platelet count (HELLP) syndrome) in women with aPL with a previous delivery for HD and/or small-for-gestational-age birth weight before 34 weeks gestation. The study was terminated early due to a low event rate and the final analysis on 33 (recruitment target was 85 women to detect a 50% risk reduction) women did not show any significant difference between aspirin alone or aspirin in combination with LMWH.

A meta-analysis comparing LMWH versus no LMWH for the prevention of recurrent placenta-mediated pregnancy complications in 848 pregnant women with a previous history of placental-mediated pregnancy complications showed a relative risk reduction of 0.52 (95% CI, 0.32–0.86) in women treated with LMWH. The meta-analysis did not confirm any reduction of early pregnancy loss (<20 weeks) in patients with prior placenta-mediated pregnancy complications, whereas a statistically non-significant reduction in late pregnancy loss (>20 weeks) was observed (7). Moreover, results from a multicentre randomized controlled trial on 150 mg aspirin daily versus placebo in 1776 pregnant women at high risk for pre-term pre-eclampsia showed aspirin to significantly reduce the risk of preeclampsia before week 34 of gestation (1.6% versus 4.3%, OR 0.38, 95th CI 0.20–0.74; p = 0.004) (8). However, one should note that the dose of aspirin trialled in the study is higher than the level commonly prescribed in many countries (75–100 mg).

The EULAR recommendation for women with aPL encourages that pregnant women with aPL should undergo foetal surveillance with Doppler ultrasonography and biometric parameters particularly in the 3rd trimester to screen for placental insufficiency and small-for-gestational-age foetuses (4). Poor flow on uterine artery Doppler is an indirect indicator for the development of placental insufficiency later in pregnancy, and in pregnant women with APS normal uterine artery blood flow between 20–24 weeks has a high negative predictive value of poor foetal outcome (3).

Case 3: Refractory obstetric APS

A 41-year-old artist is attending your pregnancy counselling clinic. She is known with APS and has a history of eight consecutive pregnancy losses before week 10. In her previous pregnancies she received either aspirin alone or a combination of aspirin and LMWH. She would like to know if there are any other treatment options as she is keen for another pregnancy.

Case discussion

The patient has been refractory to previous treatments with LDA alone and in combination with LMWH and is therefore referred to as refractory obstetric APS. The management of women with aPL or APS in pregnancy is outlined in Table 8.3.1.

There is little evidence on the treatment of women with a history of recurrent pregnancy loss despite the treatment with aspirin and LMWH. No randomized controlled trials are currently available. Agents used in refractory obstetric APS include low-dose prednisolone, intravenous immunoglobulins (IVIG), hydroxychloroquine, and statins have been suggested to potentially improve pregnancy outcomes. Low-dose oral prednisolone (10 mg daily) during the 1st trimester has been reported to improve the live birth rate in several retrospective cohorts. IVIG in addition to LDA +/- LMWH has been suggested to reduce intrauterine growth restriction, however, the treatment is costly, IVIG is invasive, and the EULAR currently only recommends its use in highly selected cases. Data on the beneficial effect of hydroxychloroquine in addition to LDA +/- LMWH on overall pregnancy outcomes and live birth rate has provided the foundation for ongoing randomized controlled trials whose results are eagerly awaited. Lastly pravastatin in addition to LDA and LMWH in women with prior aPL-related PET and intrauterine growth restriction may play a role in the prevention of placental mediated complications in these women, however, no randomized controlled trial has so far addressed the question and statins are generally not recommended during pregnancy. It is important to stress that decisions upon treatment escalation should be made together with the patient.

Taking all these factors together, in refractory cases, the most common practice if the combination of LDA and prophylactic dose heparin fails is to increase the dose of heparin to therapeutic dose, although no supporting evidence exists. Other treatment strategies may include the addition of HCQ and low-dose prednisolone, leaving the use of other approaches to very selected cases. Decisions upon treatment escalation in refractory obstetric APS should be made on a case-by-case basis and might vary in different units across the world; however, the use of low-dose prednisolone and hydroxychloroquine (<5 mg/kg) are potentially the most commonly used escalation treatments if treatment with LDA +/- LMWH fails. In patients with established diabetes mellitus or in patients at risk for gestational diabetes the addition of low-dose prednisolone should be used with caution as prednisolone is associated with the risk of developing gestational diabetes, and is known to dysregulate blood sugars. In the case of hydroxychloroquine, physicians should be cautious if a patient has known psoriasis or epilepsy (as these are general contraindications for its use as per the SmPC).

Key messages

- APS is characterized by arterial and/or venous thromboses and/or obstetric morbidity in patients persistently positive for moderate to high titres of aPL according to the current classification criteria.
- Pregnancy morbidity includes unexplained consecutive recurrent 1st trimester pregnancy loss (<10 weeks gestation), any 2nd or 3rd trimester pregnancy loss, premature birth before 34 weeks of gestation due to conditions associated with ischaemic placental dysfunction including severe pre-eclampsia, eclampsia, foetal growth restriction, and intrauterine death.
- Current treatment to prevent obstetrical morbidity is based on LDA and/or LMWH and has improved pregnancy outcomes to achieve successful live birth in >70% of pregnancies. Although hydroxychloroquine and pravastatin might further improve pregnancy outcomes, prospective clinical trials are required to confirm these findings.

Further reading

1. Miyakis S, Lockshin MD, Atsumi T, et al. International consensus statement on an update of the classification criteria for definite antiphospholipid syndrome (APS). *J Thromb Haemost.* 2006;4(2):295–306.
2. Cervera R, Serrano R, Pons-Estel GJ, et al. Morbidity and mortality in the antiphospholipid syndrome during a 10-year period: A multicentre prospective study of 1000 patients. *Ann Rheum Dis.* 2015;74(6):1011–18.
3. Schreiber K, Sciascia S, de Groot PG, et al. Antiphospholipid syndrome. *Nat Rev Dis Primers.* 2018;4:18005.
4. Andreoli L, Bertsias GK, Agmon-Levin N, et al. EULAR recommendations for women's health and the management of family planning, assisted reproduction, pregnancy and menopause in patients with systemic lupus erythematosus and/or antiphospholipid syndrome. *Ann Rheum Dis.* 2017;76(3):476–85.
5. ACOG Practice Bulletin No. 196: Thromboembolism in pregnancy. *Obstet Gynecol.* 2018 Jul;132(1):e1–e17.
6. Bates SM, Greer IA, Pabinger I, Sofaer S, Hirsh J. Venous thromboembolism, thrombophilia, antithrombotic therapy, and pregnancy: American College of Chest Physicians Evidence-Based Clinical Practice Guidelines (8th Edition). *Chest.* 2008 Jun;133(6 Suppl):844S–886S.
7. Rodger MA, Gris JC, de Vries JIP, et al. Low-molecular-weight heparin and recurrent placenta-mediated pregnancy complications: a meta-analysis of individual patient data from randomised controlled trials. *Lancet.* 2016 Nov 26;388(10060):2629–2641.
8. Rolnik DL, Wright D, Poon LC, et al. Aspirin versus Placebo in Pregnancies at High Risk for Preterm Preeclampsia. *N Engl J Med.* 2017 Aug 17;377(7):613–622.

8.4

Vasculitis in pregnancy

Megan Clowse and Jon Golenbiewski

Introduction

Outcomes in systemic vasculitis have improved dramatically, and as a result, more women with vasculitis are becoming pregnant. Problematic, however, is the paucity of information regarding pregnancy outcomes in the vasculitides, in part because of the relative infrequency of these pregnancies which precludes large collections of data.

Cohort studies include some information to guide management of Behçet's disease (BD) and Takayasu arteritis (TAK) in pregnancy. Antineutrophil cytoplasmic antibody (ANCA)-associated vasculitis (AAV), which includes granulomatosis with polyangiitis (GPA), microscopic polyangiitis (MPA), and eosinophilic granulomatosis with polyangiitis (EGPA) often affects women beyond childbearing years, but there exists a growing body of cases reported in pregnancy. Only sporadic data about pregnancy is available for more uncommon forms of disease.

Women with vasculitis have higher rates of pregnancy loss and pre-term births than the general population, likely correlating with increased disease activity (1). Although the disease course is highly variable and has the potential for complications, the majority of pregnancies in women with vasculitis that are timed to coincide with disease quiescence and managed with pregnancy-compatible medications can result in a healthy mother and child.

Takayasu arteritis (TAK)

Case 1: Patient with TAK

A 31-year-old female with past medical history of hypertension was diagnosed with TAK at age 28 with disease manifestations of right subclavian artery stenosis, mild aortic regurgitation, and left carotid artery stenosis. She had one previous pregnancy at age 30 that was complicated by a hypertensive emergency at 35 weeks, resulting in an emergency Caesarean section (CS). The baby was small for gestational age but was otherwise healthy. Her disease has been quiet for the past 6 months on prednisone, methotrexate, and infliximab. She desires to become pregnant and seeks rheumatological opinion prior to attempting conception.

On physical examination she is afebrile with a normal heart rate and body mass index of 27. Blood pressure in the right arm is 102/78 and 142/90 in the left arm. Right lower extremity blood pressure is 138/82 and the left lower extremity 142/90. Her right upper extremity distal pulse is diminished, with remaining pulses strong and equal throughout. There is a soft diastolic murmur over the aortic valve and bruits over the left carotid artery and right axilla. She is not currently taking antihypertensive medications.

Effect of disease on pregnancy

TAK is a large vessel vasculitis defined by arterial stenoses and aneurysmal dilatations of the aorta and its branches in an asymmetric distribution, most commonly diagnosed in women less than age 40. While most pregnancies are successful, women with TAK can experience complications, in particular, during the peripartum period (2). Severe hypertension and pre-eclampsia are among the most common complications, having affected 43% of pregnancies reported in the literature, markedly higher than the general population (3). Pre-eclampsia in TAK has a greater association with stillbirth than in the general population (3).

Effect of pregnancy on disease

TAK does not flare during pregnancy often, with only seven flares having been reported in 214 pregnancies in the literature (3).

Management

Acute phase reactants should be used to monitor for inflammation, see Box 8.4.1; the C-reactive protein (CRP) can be a somewhat more reliable measure of inflammation, as the erythrocyte sedimentation rate (ESR) is universally elevated in all pregnant patients (4). It must be recognized, however, that active TAK is not always associated with elevated acute phase reactants, and often relies on new symptoms or changes on physical examination. Constitutional symptoms, signs of ischaemia, or new murmurs or bruits on examination can indicate active disease. Imaging can identify vascular changes, with magnetic resonance imaging (MRI) being preferable to avoid radiation exposure and for improved imaging of blood vessels and blood vessel walls.

Blood pressure monitoring of all four extremities should routinely be performed. Peripheral pressures can be inaccurate in TAK, and in certain situations may need to be monitored through invasive means (4). Poorly controlled blood pressure can predispose to worsening of aortic aneurysms, dissection, and aortic insufficiency; this concern is elevated in pregnancy, as it normally results in an increase in plasma volume. Vascular intervention on aneurysms and severe stenoses should occur ideally prior to becoming pregnant during periods of low disease activity.

Vaginal delivery can increase blood pressure, and CS may be a reasonable choice in those with uncontrolled hypertension (3). Pain control is especially important to avoid increases in blood pressure. Conversely, hypotension should be avoided, as general anaesthesia or spinal block can result in decreased lower extremity perfusion in patients with stenoses. Some experts recommend epidural anaesthesia be used in cases which require CS (4), and regional anaesthesia should be used when possible (3). Vascular intervention should be reserved only for emergency situations.

Box 8.4.1 Takayasu arteritis key points

Monitoring:
- Prior to pregnancy, assess degree of vascular disease through symptoms, examination, and imaging.
- Echocardiogram should be performed to assess for aortic dilatation and regurgitation.
- Critical stenosis, aneurysmal dilatation, and aortic regurgitation should be evaluated by a vascular specialist, with an emphasis on planned intervention prior to pregnancy.
- Blood pressure should be checked and documented in all four extremities at each visit and correlated with available imaging to determine which limb is most reflective of the true blood pressure. In cases where this cannot be determined, and there is question of ongoing hypertension, invasive monitoring may be needed.

Management points:
- Blood pressure should be managed aggressively, with careful attention to avoid hypotension.
- CS should be considered in patients with tenuous blood pressures, with epidural or regional anaesthesia, preferred to avoid hypotension.
- Decreases in blood pressure in specific limbs could be reflective of active disease and progressive stenosis.
- Consult with anaesthesia for peripartum management.

Medications:
- Pregnancy-compatible medications: TNF inhibitors, azathioprine, corticosteroids (use sparingly).
- For severe disease: high-dose steroids, tocilizumab (limited safety data), Cyclophosphamide in the 2nd or 3rd trimester, if no other options.

Therapy in pregnancy

Steroids should be used sparingly and, when possible, replaced with pregnancy-compatible immunosuppressants including azathioprine and TNF inhibitors. Methotrexate should be stopped prior to conception (see Chapter 3.1). Tocilizumab has been used in TAK, although there is limited data about its safety in pregnancy. Antihypertensive therapy should be maximized in conjunction with the obstetric team.

Behçet's Disease (BD)

Case 2: Patient with BD desires pregnancy

A 25-year-old female with BD discovered she is 8 weeks pregnant. She has no prior pregnancies or comorbidities. She was diagnosed with BD 2 years prior with disease characterized by recurrent aphthous ulcers, inflammatory arthritis, and superficial thrombophlebitis. She had an acute deep vein thrombosis (DVT) 1 year ago which was treated with anticoagulation for 6 months. She is currently taking 0.6 mg of colchicine daily, but still has episodic flares of ulcers and polyarticular arthritis for which she takes prednisone about 3 days per month. On examination vital signs are normal, with a body mass index of 30. There is evidence of synovitis involving the right wrist and right 2nd proximal interphalangeal (PIP) joint. She has scattered pustules on the proximal thighs and no evidence of vasculitis involving the skin. She would like to discuss treatment options during pregnancy, including the role for anticoagulation given her prior history of DVT.

Effect of disease on pregnancy

BD is a multisystem vasculitis that affects arteries and veins of variable size, resulting in a combination of oral and/or vaginal ulcers, skin involvement, inflammatory arthritis, thrombosis, pulmonary artery aneurysms, gastrointestinal tract involvement, and CNS vasculitis in extreme cases. For women with mild-moderate disease, pregnancy outcomes are comparable to the general population (2), with overall low rates of hypertension, pre-eclampsia, pre-term delivery, and foetal loss (3). Pregnant patients with BD are at increased risk of DVT, considering both conditions are associated with thrombosis. There is very limited data on pregnancies in women with severe BD.

Effect of pregnancy on disease

Disease tends to improve during pregnancy, reported in up to 60% of cases in a large systematic review (3). Flares may occur during pregnancy, most commonly being mucocutaneous ulcerations or arthritis (4).

Management

Corticosteroids, azathioprine, colchicine, ciclosporin, and tumour necrosis factor (TNF) inhibitors can all be utilized (see also Box 8.4.2 and Chapter 3.1). Oral and vaginal ulcers can be treated with topical steroids or colchicine. Continuing colchicine for the duration of pregnancy may allow for less corticosteroid exposure (2). Severe manifestations mid-pregnancy require assessment of the risks versus benefits of cyclophosphamide, which can be used in the 2nd and 3rd trimesters. There is some increased risk for pregnancy loss with cyclophosphamide use during pregnancy, although it is difficult to determine if this is related to cyclophosphamide itself versus the effects of severe, active disease on the pregnancy.

Women with BD should be monitored closely for thrombosis, especially in the 6 weeks following delivery. Therapeutic anticoagulation should be prescribed in patients with prior DVT; preventive anticoagulation is not required in patients without a prior thrombotic event, but aspirin may be used. Pulmonary artery aneurysm is a known, but rare, complication of BD and should be considered in pregnancy if a woman with BD has abrupt onset of dyspnea or haemoptysis; acute evaluation is required with a preference for MRI, though other modalities may be needed for specific patients that pose manageable risks in pregnancy.

Box 8.4.2 Behçet's disease key points

Monitoring:
- Assess symptoms prior to and during pregnancy.
- Monitor for symptoms of DVT.

Management points:
- Assess hypercoagulable risk; consider prophylactic anticoagulation if prior thrombosis.
- Pulmonary artery aneurysm should be considered in patients with chest pain, shortness of breath, haemoptysis.

Medications:
- Continuation of colchicine throughout disease may decrease steroid exposure and improve disease control.
- Pregnancy-compatible medications: azathioprine, cyclosporin, tacrolimus, TNF inhibitors, corticosteroids (use sparingly).
- For severe disease: high-dose steroids, cyclophosphamide in the 2nd or 3rd trimester, if no other options.

ANCA-associated vasculitis

Case 3: Patient with granulomatosis polyangiitis (GPA) planning pregnancy

A 37-year-old female with GPA desires to become pregnant. Her disease was diagnosed 8 years prior, with initial presentation of chronic sinusitis, small vessel vasculitis of the skin, cavitary lung involvement, and rapidly progressive glomerulonephritis that required temporary haemodialysis. She had full recovery of renal function after being treated with high-dose methylprednisolone and induction therapy with rituximab. She had an excellent response to rituximab and was on maintenance therapy with azathioprine 100 mg daily while weaning off prednisone. This was decreased to 50 mg daily after 2 years of disease quiescence.

While in remission the patient had two pregnancies that both resulted in pre-term delivery (one at 31 weeks, the other at 35 weeks). She remained on azathioprine until 6 months prior to presentation, during which her disease flared with biopsy proven active pauci-immune necrotizing crescentic glomerulonephritis. She again received rituximab with high-dose methylprednisolone. Her physical examination is normal and she has no symptoms to suggest active disease after rituximab induction. There has been normalization of her creatinine and urine protein to creatinine ratio, with a bland urine sediment on follow-up. She is currently due for another dose of rituximab. She would like to know if it is safe to take rituximab while pregnant and while breastfeeding.

Effect of disease on pregnancy

ANCA-associated vasculitis (AAV) refers to a group of small vessel vasculitides (GPA, MPA, and EGPA) that are less commonly described in pregnancy, given the typical older age of onset and prior heavy reliance on high-doses of cyclophosphamide that impaired fertility. GPA and MPA commonly manifest with pulmonary and renal disease, whereas EGPA is defined by allergic rhinosinusitis, asthma, and small vessel vasculitis that less commonly involves the kidneys. Women with active disease at conception and those with new disease during pregnancy are at high risk for poor outcomes related to maternal complications and death (3). There is an increased risk of premature delivery in GPA, having been reported in 35% of pregnancies, with the risk increased by active disease (3). Pre-term birth is the most common complication of EGPA, similar to GPA (2).

Effect of pregnancy on disease

Flares are common, even with disease quiescence during conception, with 40% of patients (12 out of 30) having flares amongst reported cases in the literature (3). Monitoring should include assessment of renal function and urinalysis for the development of glomerulonephritis, which can be difficult to differentiate from pre-eclampsia. Additionally, CRP levels and ANCA titres can be monitored in patients who are known to have levels that correlate with disease. A rapid worsening of breathing in the setting of active disease should lead one to consider diffuse alveolar haemorrhage or other serious cardiopulmonary pathology.

In EGPA, patients with severe asthma can have worsening outcomes due to loss of lung capacity associated with pregnancy (4) and should be co-managed with pulmonology. Cardiac involvement can occur in EGPA; an echocardiogram should be obtained when symptoms are suggestive of heart failure. Carpal tunnel syndrome is a common side effect of pregnancy, but if hand numbness and weakness occurs, AAV-related neuropathy can be considered; electromyography may prove helpful in distinguishing these entities.

Management

Rituximab has become the gold standard in the treatment of AAV in young patients (see Box 8.4.3). Data suggests that conception in the months following rituximab infusion does not increase the risk for pregnancy loss or birth defects, suggesting dosing rituximab prior to conception may be a valid method for achieving disease control prior to and during pregnancy (2). Rituximab crosses the placenta starting around week 16, with increasing transfer closer to delivery, which can result in B cell depletion in infants (3). About half of infants exposed in the latter half of pregnancy to maternal rituximab will have no B cells at birth; despite this, limited data shows no major increased infectious risk to the newborn to date.

If rituximab is required in pregnancy, it is recommended to dose prior to 16 weeks gestation. In general, it would be advisable to avoid rituximab in cases of mild disease that can be controlled with azathioprine and/or low-dose corticosteroids. However, it should be utilized in cases of severe, organ-threatening disease (see following).

Box 8.4.3 ANCA-associated vasculitis key points

Monitoring:

- ANCA titres should be monitored in patients with levels corresponding to disease activity.
- Urinalysis should be monitored for an active sediment, suggestive of glomerulonephritis.

Management points:
- Asthma in EGPA should be co-managed with assistance of pulmonology.
- Hypertension needs to be carefully controlled.
- Monitor for thrombosis in pregnancy.

Medications:
- Pregnancy-compatible medications: azathioprine, cyclosporin, tacrolimus, corticosteroids (use sparingly).
- Consider rituximab prior to conception to control vasculitis; can dose in the 1st half of pregnancy and following delivery. Avoid in 2nd half of pregnancy. Rituximab should not interfere with breastfeeding.
- For severe disease: high-dose steroids, cyclophosphamide in the 2nd or 3rd trimester, if no other options.

Because rituximab is an IgG1 antibody and a very large molecule, there is believed to be extremely limited transfer in breastmilk at levels that would not be toxic to the nursing infant (5).

Treatment for a severe flare during pregnancy is more challenging. As in the non-pregnant patient, corticosteroids should be used to gain disease control, given its rapid onset of action and effective suppression of disease. In severe, organ-threatening disease, rituximab could be used given the low risks known to date for adverse foetal effects compared to the high potential for both maternal and foetal complications associated with active disease. Cyclophosphamide can be given in the 2nd and 3rd trimesters for life-threatening disease as well (4). Plasma exchange has been used in pregnancy, although its benefit for vasculitis is now being questioned. Other treatments include azathioprine and steroids. The safety of mepolizumab, an IL-5 inhibitor sometimes used for EGPA, is unknown in pregnancy and its use is not recommended. There is an increased risk of thrombosis in AAV, and anticoagulation is indicated in women with a prior thrombotic event. In women who require high doses of immunosuppression, dapsone should be considered for pneumocystis prophylaxis.

Key messages

- Pregnancies in systemic vasculitis are rare, with the majority of data coming from cohort studies and case reports.

- In general, women with vasculitis in pregnancy have good maternal and foetal outcomes when pregnancy is well-timed and disease is controlled with pregnancy-compatible immunosuppressive medications that are continued for the duration of pregnancy.
- Women with vasculitis should be monitored closely as part of a multidisciplinary team that includes maternal foetal medicine, amongst others.

Further reading

1. Clowse ME, et al. Pregnancy outcomes among patients with vasculitis. *Arthritis Care Res* (Hoboken). 2013;65(8):1370–4.
2. Machen L, ME Clowse. Vasculitis and pregnancy. *Rheum Dis Clin North Am.* 2017;43(2):239–47.
3. Gatto M, et al. Pregnancy and vasculitis: A systematic review of the literature. *Autoimmun Rev.* 2012;11(6–7):A447–59.
4. Seo P. Pregnancy and vasculitis. *Rheum Dis Clin North Am.* 2007;33(2):299–317.
5. Bragnes Y., et al. Low level of Rituximab in human breast milk in a patient treated during lactation. *Rheumatology* (Oxford). 2017;56(6):1047–8.

8.5

Systemic sclerosis

Eliza Chakravarty

Introduction

Systemic sclerosis (SSc) is a progressive autoimmune disease that is characterized by a non-inflammatory vasculopathy as well as fibrosis of the skin and vital organs. It is divided into two subsets based on the extent of cutaneous involvement (diffuse vs limited cutaneous SSc). Although the prevalence of different organ involvement varies between the two subsets, all are at potential risk for the development of digital necrosis and gangrene, intestinal malabsorption, cardiac and pulmonary fibrosis, scleroderma renal crisis (SRC), and pulmonary arterial hypertension (PAH). Unlike other autoimmune diseases for which immunosuppressive regimens have demonstrated success in ameliorating active inflammatory disease, SSc has a paucity of true disease-modifying agents. Therapies for SSc are mostly directed at managing symptoms with vasodilators, angiotensin-renin antagonists, proton pump inhibitors, and immunosuppressives in the case of pulmonary fibrosis. The age of onset of SSc is generally after the childbearing years and most women have completed their families prior to diagnosis and are usually not pursuing future pregnancies. Because SSc has a significantly lower prevalence than other autoimmune disease and the age of onset is often in the 4th and 5th decade, the literature experience describing pregnancy outcomes is much more sparse than with more common autoimmune diseases that often present earlier in life.

Because of the severity of many internal organ manifestations of SSc, maternal health may be at risk if medications with teratogenic potential must be discontinued for a pregnancy for which no safer options exist. Pre-conception counselling is critical to review an individual woman's disease manifestations, degree of damage, and required medications before a woman makes a decision regarding proceeding with a pregnancy. In contrast, those with skin-predominant disease who have little to no organ involvement may be at lower risk for pregnancy complications involving mother and baby.

Cutaneous disease

Progression of underlying cutaneous fibrosis is uncommon during pregnancy, even in women with diffuse cutaneous SSc. In most studies, the majority of women have no significant change in the degree of skin thickening during their pregnancy, with a smaller proportion experiencing either improvement or worsening of skin disease.

Furthermore, the degree of cutaneous involvement has not been associated with adverse pregnancy outcomes.

Vascular disease

Case 1: Patient with diffuse cutaneous SSc planning pregnancy

A 33-year-old woman with a 6-year history of diffuse cutaneous systemic sclerosis (dcSSc) mentions during routine follow-up that she wants to become pregnant for the first time. She has diffuse skin involvement involving her face, chest, forearms, and abdomen that has resulted in contractures over several proximal interphalangeal joints and reduced oral aperture. She has a 10-year history of Raynaud's disease with digital ulcerations and loss of digital pulp. She has had routine monitoring by echocardiogram and pulmonary function tests that have not shown evidence of pulmonary arterial hypertension (PAH). She has no history of scleroderma renal crisis (SRC) or other internal organ involvement. She is on a stable regimen of amlodipine and omeprazole. Physical examination shows matted telangiectasias on her face and oropharynx, diffuse skin thickening, mild loss of digital pulp on most fingers, and two ulcers on her finger tips that are in the process of healing. She is concerned about what medications she can take during her pregnancy and if her ulcerations will worsen.

Case discussion

Raynaud's disease is an extremely common manifestation of both diffuse and limited cutaneous SSc, with digital ulcerations and digital gangrene from inadequate blood supply as an unfortunate, but much less common, complication of the disease. The pathophysiology of Raynaud's and digital gangrene in scleroderma patients is a non-inflammatory vasculopathy involving progressive intimal fibrosis of the arterial walls. Depending on the degree of symptoms and evidence of arterial insufficiency, various vasodilators are used to maximize blood flow to the digits. These include: calcium channel blockers, topical nitrates, anticoagulants, endothelin receptor antagonists, phosphodiesterase-type 5 inhibitors, and prostacyclins. Non-pharmacological interventions included physical warming of trunk and digits, digital sympathectomy, and amputation for unattenuated and progressive gangrene.

Fortunately, some of the normal physiological changes occurring during pregnancy can ameliorate or attenuate Raynaud's disease and related vasculopathy. Beginning in the first weeks of gestation, maternal plasma volume increases by approximately 50% to accommodate the high-volume perfusion required by the placenta. The increased plasma volume combined with reduced systemic vascular resistance can lead to improved perfusion of the digits with resulting improvements in both Raynaud's symptoms and digital ulcers. Digital gangrene occurring during pregnancy is extremely rare, and often associated with concomitant beta blocker therapy or other pregnancy complications (e.g. pregnancy induced hypertension). Therefore, pharmacological therapy for peripheral vasculopathy in SSc may not be as intensive as when a woman is not pregnant. Calcium channel blockers have not been shown to be teratogenic, and are considered compatible with pregnancy. They may be continued throughout pregnancy in women using them prior to conception, and can be safely added during pregnancy for management of hypertension as well as symptomatic Raynaud's. Patients should be advised that the vasodilation associated with calcium channel blockers in the setting of reduced systemic resistance could lead to symptomatic hypotension during pregnancy, so blood pressure should be monitored and the dose titrated appropriately. Similarly, for more severe cases of vasculopathy and refractory digital ulcers, sildenafil can be used during pregnancy, as can low-dose aspirin, and heparin products. Endothelin receptor antagonists should be avoided in pregnancy as they may adversely affect foetal vascular development. Therefore, women receiving these agents should switch to calcium channel blockers, sildenafil, or prostacyclins prior to or as soon as pregnancy is discovered. Prostacyclin analogues can be used for emergency treatment of gangrene during pregnancy.

Pulmonary arterial hypertension

Pulmonary arterial hypertension (PAH) is a well-known vascular complication affecting up to 20% of SSc patients. It occurs more frequently in limited cutaneous SSc than diffuse cutaneous disease, but both subsets are at risk for the condition. PAH is among the most severe manifestations of SSc, even in the non-pregnant patient, and is associated with high morbidity and markedly decreased survival. Because the pathology of PAH is a fixed and progressive vasculopathy of the pulmonary arteries, the excess blood volume associated with normal pregnancies places the mother at even higher risk of death from PAH. Therefore, PAH is one of the comorbidities of SSc for which pregnancy is strongly contraindicated. If a woman with known SSc is considering a future pregnancy, screening for subclinical PAH is highly recommended and counselling provided to those with evidence of PAH. Women with symptomatic PAH should be strongly discouraged against pregnancy and to consider long-acting or permanent forms of contraception. See Chapter 2.2 for further discussion of PAH during pregnancy.

Scleroderma renal crisis

Case 2: Patient with scleroderma renal crisis

A 27-year-old woman with a 3-year history of dcSSc presents for routine follow-up at 16 weeks' gestation of her first pregnancy. Prior to becoming pregnant, disease manifestations included progressive cutaneous sclerosis involving both arms, feet, back, abdomen, and face, with reduced oral aperture and matted telangiectasias. She had Raynaud's with digital ulcers in the past, but these have improved since pregnancy. She did not have any history of pulmonary, cardiac, or renal disease. Pre-pregnancy medications included a proton pump inhibitor for gastric reflux and a calcium channel blocker for Raynaud's. A multivitamin was added in anticipation of a pregnancy. At her week 16 visit, she endorsed increased fatigue and malaise, which she attributed to pregnancy. On physical examination, she was found to have an elevated blood pressure of

183/96 and mild oedema in her ankles. Laboratory samples drawn at that visit showed a drop in haemoglobin, new thrombocytopenia with a platelet count of 55,000, doubling of serum creatinine, and urinalysis showing proteinuria and red blood cells. She was admitted to the hospital for further management. Repeat laboratory studies were unchanged. A renal biopsy was felt to be of too high risk, and was therefore not performed.

Case discussion

This situation is a medical emergency; and the differential diagnosis in this setting is pre-eclampsia or SRC. Because she is less than 20 weeks' gestation, pre-eclampsia is less likely. Additionally, the definitive treatment for pre-eclampsia is delivery of the foetus and placenta, which would result in termination of her pre-viable pregnancy. SRC is the most likely underlying cause of this patient's sudden deterioration, with evidence of new severe hypertension, renal dysfunction, and possible haemolytic anaemia. She is at high risk for SRC given she is within 5 years of a diagnosis of dcSSc with progressive cutaneous disease. Specific autoantibody patterns, although they can be helpful in predicting patients who may be at higher risk for later development of SRC, will not be able to distinguish existing SRC from other causes of microangiopathy. Because use of high-dose corticosteroids is a known risk factor for the development of SRC and may contribute to its worsening, it is important to avoid administration of corticosteroids in this case, even while the exact diagnosis is unknown.

The main therapy for SRC in the non-pregnant patient is angiotensin-converting enzyme inhibitors (ACE-I) or angiotensin-receptor blockers (ARB) as the pathology is thought to be activation of the renin-angiotensin-aldosterone system. Both ACE-I and ARBs are generally contraindicated during pregnancy because of associations with small increases in congenital anomalies following 1st trimester exposure, as well as significantly increased risks (10–20%) of renal papillary atrophy with 2nd and 3rd trimester exposure. Therefore, they should not be used during pregnancy if other classes of medications can be used that are more compatible with pregnancy. However, in the case of SRC, other anti-hypertensive medications have not been shown to have benefit in SRC, and the only option to reverse the condition and protect the life and health of the mother (and subsequently, the foetus) is to promptly initiate an angiotensin-converting enzyme (ACE) at the earliest suspicion of SRC, despite the trimester of pregnancy. It is recommended that captopril be used because of its short half-life and ability to titrate rapidly to achieve control of blood pressure and renal function. Patients should be hospitalized for close blood pressure and urinary output monitoring. Captopril doses can start as low as 12.5 mg orally, and titrated upward every 8 hours to achieve a blood pressure of 120/70 within 72 hours. Response to ACE-I can be seen within a short time frame, whereas untreated disease can also progress rapidly to anuric renal failure, foetal demise, and even maternal death. Thus, when SRC is suspected, it is recommended to proceed first with ACE-I as quickly as possible, then to consider other causes of microangiopathy if symptoms persist or worsen. Studies have not identified a particular embryopathy associated with 1st trimester use of ACE or ARB medications; an overall increase in congenital anomalies with 1st trimester exposure is similar to what is seen in hypertensive women treated with other anti-hypertensive agents. Use in later tri-mesters of pregnancy, however, is associated with foetal renal failure, renal dys-plasia, oligohydramnios, and pulmonary hypoplasia, although it is not clear if such manifestations are due to direct foetotoxicity or hypoperfusion. Nonetheless, the risks of foetopathy with use of ACE-I or ARB must be weighed against the high risk of progressive morbidity and possible mortality of the mother and subsequent pregnancy loss.

Intrauterine growth restriction

Because vasculopathy can be such a prominent feature of both diffuse and limited cutaneous SSc, the effects of abnormalities of placental vasculature on the growing foetus are of obvious concern. Therefore, it is not surprising that rates of both pre-term delivery and small-for-gestational-age neonates are elevated in SSc patients compared to the general obstetric population in nearly all studies published to date. For the most part, these perinatal complications were usually mild to moderate, and the incidence of severe pre-term delivery or low birth rate infants leading to perinatal morbidity and mortality remains low. There are few reports describing placental pathology in women with SSc. When performed, these often show vasculopathic changes similar to what is seen in placentas of women with pregnancy-induced hypertension, and can occur even in pregnancies with uncomplicated outcomes. Elevated rates of pre-eclampsia have generally not been seen in SSc pregnancies, further suggesting that placental vas-cular disease is one that develops later during gestation rather than during early plac-entation and spiral artery development.

Although seen with more frequency than in otherwise healthy women, complica-tions of placental vasculopathy (intrauterine growth restriction, premature delivery) are most commonly of mild to moderate severity and overall pregnancy outcomes are favourable. Increase surveillance of foetal growth during the latter half of preg-nancy may be warranted, but specific therapeutic interventions to treat growth re-striction have not be identified. Severe placental compromise leading to intrauterine or neonatal death remain very rare, and women with stable, non-organ-threatening SSc should not be discouraged from pregnancy solely out of fear of increased adverse pregnancy outcomes.

Key messages

- The onset of SSc is commonly in the 4th and 5th decade of life, long after women have completed their families.
- Common symptoms of SSc, including cutaneous fibrosis and Raynaud's phe-nomenon, do not worsen, and often improve symptomatically during pregnancy.
- Moderate to severe interstitial lung disease and PAH are relative contraindica-tions to pregnancy because of significantly increased risk of maternal morbidity and mortality.
- The onset of SRC during pregnancy necessitates the use of ACE-I or ARB, despite their association with teratogenicity and foetopathy.

- Placental vasculopathy in SSc mirrors disease-related vasculopathy. Risks of pre-eclampsia are generally not elevated, but intrauterine growth restriction does occur during the later months of pregnancy because of non-inflammatory placental vasculopathy.

Further reading

1. Allanore Y, Denton CP, Krieg T, Cornelisse P, Rosenberg D, Schwierin B, Matucci-Cerinic M. DUO Investigators. Clinical characteristics and predictors of gangrene in patients with systemic sclerosis and digital ulcers in the Digital Ulcer Outcome Registry: A prospective, observational cohort. *Ann Rheum Dis.* 2016;75(9):1736–40.
2. da Silva Ferreira RD, Negrini R, Bernardo WM, Simões R, Piato S. The effects of sildenafil in maternal and fetal outcomes in pregnancy: A systematic review and meta-analysis. *PLoS One.* 2019;14(7):e0219732. doi: 10.1371/journal.pone.0219732. eCollection 2019.
3. Nadeem S, Hashmat S, Defreitas MJ, Westreich KD, Shatat IF, Selewski DT, et al. Renin angiotensin system blocker fetopathy: A midwest pediatric nephrology consortium report. *J Pediatr.* 2015 Oct;167(4):881–5. doi: 10.1016/j.jpeds.2015.05.045. Epub 2015 Jun 27.
4. Sobanski V, Launay D, Depret S, Ducloy-Bouthors AS, Hachulla E. Special considerations in pregnant systemic sclerosis patients. *Exp Rev Clin Immunol.* 2016;12:1161–73.
5. Quan A. Fetopathy associated with exposure to angiotensin converting enzyme inhibitors and angiotension receptor antagonists. *Early Hum Dev.* 2006;82(1):23–8.

8.6
Myositis and pregnancy

Muhammad Shipa and David Isenberg

Introduction

Idiopathic inflammatory myositis (IIM) comprise a group of diseases of unknown cause resulting in muscle inflammation and subsequent muscle weakness. Inflammatory myositis (IM) cases are rare, with an incidence of 5–10 cases per million people, and mainly develop in women (female:male = 2–3:1) often after the age of 40, when women are less likely to become pregnant. Only 14% of myositis patients develop the disease before or during the childbearing years (1). Reports on pregnancies in myositis patients are very rare and consist mainly of case reports and small series collected over several decades with variance in patient characteristics and management. Thus the paucity of cases makes it hard to offer confident advice to the patient about pregnancy outcome. We will discuss a few of our challenging patients here, who have been seen over the last 20 years.

Case 1: Effect of myositis on pregnancy and vice versa

A 28-year-old Indian female was diagnosed with polymyositis at age 25. Three years ago, she presented with proximal muscle weakness of upper and lower limb with raised creatine kinase (CK). There was no skin rash, swallowing or breathing difficulties, or joint pain. Her antinuclear antibody (ANA), extractable nuclear antibody (ENA), anti-double stranded DNA (ds-DNA) antibodies, and myositis specific antibodies were negative. Subsequent muscle biopsy was consistent with polymyositis. She had no past medical history or significant family history. She was a smoker (average 20/day for 8 years) and drank socially. Her body mass index (BMI) was 24. She was treated with prednisolone (current dose 2.5 mg daily), azathioprine (current dose 75 mg/day), and had a course of intravenous immunoglobulin (IVIG) 3 years ago. She has been in remission for 3 years. She is now getting married. She is very concerned about her future pregnancy (nulliparous) and wants to know the effect of myositis on fertility, pregnancy, and baby, along with risk of myositis flare in pregnancy, and its inheritance.

Case discussion

Fertility in women with inflammatory myositis

The issue of fertility is difficult to address as data are limited due to the relatively late onset of disease and the general advice to use contraception if a patient is on mycophenolate or methotrexate (as these drugs should be avoided during pregnancy) (2) (see Chapter 3.1). Currently, only two studies have addressed the issue of fertility in detail (3, 4). One suggested a slight reduction in the fertility rate, but the other found no difference compared to the general population. However, as the sample size in both studies was very small, definitive conclusions are hard to reach.

Pregnancy outcome with pre-existing myositis

Active myositis can cause a serious outcome for the pregnancy. The summary of reported 74 pregnancies of 56 patients [dermatomyositis (DM) 32, juvenile dermatomyositis (JDM) 5, polymyositis (PM) 19] published between 1938–2018, is shown in Table 8.6.1. Of these, myositis flared in 15 pregnancies and seven had active disease when they became pregnant. Clearly pregnancies associated with active disease showed a higher rate of foetal deaths (31.8% in the active myositis group compared to 7.7% of inactive myositis; $p<0.05$). Notably, most of the complications in inactive disease were observed before 1984. Perivillous fibrin deposits are a rare but serious condition, whose exact aetiology is not known, but may develop in various autoimmune diseases including lupus and antiphospholipid antibody syndrome. This condition is characterized by diffuse fibrin deposits in the intra-villous space which can lead to intrauterine foetal death, intrauterine growth restriction (IUGR), and prematurity. There are five reported cases of myositis associated perivillous fibrin deposits; four of them subsequently involved foetal death (5–9). Interestingly, three of these patients were associated with an anti-synthetase antibody (aSS). Thus, aSS patients may be at a higher

Table 8.6.1 Outcome of pregnancies in women with active versus inactive myositis

Details of the pregnancies (n = 74)*	Disease activity during pregnancy	
	Active (n = 22)	Inactive (n = 52)
Duration of remission	few months to 5 years	10 months to 5 years (but incomplete data)
Age at onset of disease	20–40 years	22–42 years

Pregnancy outcomes	5 premature births
	1 IUGR**
	5 abortions
	1 stillbirth
	1 neonatal death
		1 premature birth
		3 spontaneous abortions
		   (reported before 1984)
		1 neonatal death (reported
		   before 1984)
		1 emergency Caesarean
		   section
		2 elective abortions

	7 total foetal deaths$	6 total foetal deaths$

*The n=74 figure is derived from a literature search; the most important of these references are shown in the literature list.

**IUGR = Intrauterine growth retardation.

$ Sum of abortions, stillbirths and neonatal death.

risk of developing these complications. There are reported cases of successful treatment of this condition with low-molecular-weight heparin and low-dose aspirin (10); which raises the possibility that anticoagulation may have a role, especially in those who had a prior pregnancy loss associated with perivillous fibrin deposits.

In contrast to these data, more recent reports describe fewer reported cases of foetal death. A recent observational study (11) reviewed 853 patients with DM/PM which did not suggest any differences in rates of premature rupture of membrane (PROM) or Caesarean section in patients with DM/PM compared with controls. The authors noted an increased risk of IUGR (3.1% compared to 1.4%; p = 0.05). Patients with DM/PM were more likely to have hypertensive disorders of pregnancy such as gestational hypertension, pre-eclampsia, and eclampsia (20.9% of DM/PM patients compared with 7.4% of controls; p <0.001). Moreover, patients of African-American origin and those with diabetes had an increased risk of hypertensive disorders. However, it is not clear whether the risk increases with active disease or not and the dose of steroid was not taken into consideration.

Due to the paucity of data comparing pregnancy outcome in myositis patients with matched normal populations, definitive conclusions are hard to determine.

Considering neonatal outcomes, none of the reported cases appeared to describe neonatal myositis in the newborn. In general, the neonatal outcome is good; one of the neonatal deaths was associated with a twin pregnancy.

Myositis flares during pregnancy

Several case reports and case series have reported an increased risk of flare during pregnancies. In the sparse existing literature 15 patients have been reported to have had flare out of 74 pregnancies (20%). Five patients flared in the 2nd trimester, three in the 3rd trimester, and in the other seven the onset was unclear. Two of these pregnancies were complicated by pre-eclampsia. However, more recent case reports do not support such a high rate of flare (one case series suggested it may be only 5%) (12–14), that supports the present treatment strategies which are different compared to old cases where patients often were not treated or undertreated in pregnancy and where pregnancy planning at a time of remission before conception was not required.

Inheritance

Although some genes (e.g. human leukocyte antigen 8.1 ancestral haplotype alleles) (15) have been linked to an increase in the susceptibility of the offspring, currently there is no clear evidence that risk of subsequent inflammatory myositis will be higher in the offspring.

In our case the patient is concerned about her future pregnancy and the possible effect of her myositis on fertility, pregnancy and the baby, and the risk for inheritance. In summary there are too few data to provide scientific robust evidence regarding any of her concerns. Therefore, it is important to follow her regularly during pregnancy and to liaise with her midwife and obstetrician. She would be classified as a high-risk pregnancy and a multidisciplinary team approach for the follow-up during pregnancy is extremely important.

Case 2: Onset of myositis during pregnancy

A 29-year-old African woman was referred to rheumatology from gynaecology as she had rash and weakness. She was 8 weeks pregnant (primigravida). She had proximal muscle weakness in her upper and lower limbs and the rash was consistent with DM. She had no swallowing problem or respiratory symptoms. Her CK was 8000 IU/L, Anti-MDA-5 (autoantibodies against melanoma differentiation-associated antibody) positive, but her ANA and anti-ds-DNA and ENA were negative. Muscle biopsy confirmed DM. Although anti-MDA-5 associated DM carries a high risk of lung involvement, she had no lung involvement at that point. Her past medical history included childhood asthma for which she was not on any inhalers as it was well controlled. Her BMI was 26. She never smoked but used to drink 1–2 glasses of wine once or twice per week before the pregnancy. Her family history revealed nothing of significance. She was treated with oral prednisolone (started on 40 mg once daily) along with azathioprine (100 mg daily). Eight weeks later she presented to the emergency department with difficulties of breathing with a dry cough (she was now 16 weeks pregnant). She also noted deterioration of her muscle strength. Fever, sputum, haemoptysis, chest pain, and pleurisy were absent. Her respiratory rate was 32, pulse rate 92 beats per minute; oxygen saturation was 90% on room air. On examination she had bi-basal end inspiratory crackles, JVP was not raised, and there was no pedal oedema. Blood gas analysis suggested type 1 respiratory failure; however she did not require any ventilator support other than oxygen. Urgent chest x-ray suggested marked loss of volume and diffuse ground-glass opacities, especially in the lower lung fields. Urgent blood tests showed rising CK and raised C-reactive protein. Rapidly progressive interstitial lung disease (RILD) was suspected. She was started on intravenous (IV) methylprednisolone (500 mg/day IV for 3 days) and empirical antibiotics. Bronchoalveolar lavage (BAL) excluded infection. Subsequently she was also started on oral prednisolone 20 mg/day for 2 weeks and ciclosporin 2.5 mg/kg body weight. At that point she had a viable pregnancy. After 4 weeks (now 20 weeks pregnant), her breathing deteriorated again with increasing oxygen demand and progression of ground-glass opacities on chest x-ray. Unfortunately she had to be intubated. She was given IVIG 2 mg/kg in divided dose and rituximab 1 g × 2, 2 weeks apart. These measures improved of her clinical condition and she was managed during the rest of her pregnancy on reducing doses of prednisolone and ciclosporin. Despite IUGR complicating her pregnancy, she went on to have an uncomplicated elective Caesarean section and delivered a healthy newborn.

Case discussion

Myositis may start before, during, or even after the pregnancy is completed. The literature suggests that the onset during pregnancy (1st trimester) is more common than in the puerperal period.

Pregnancy outcome with disease onset during pregnancy

To date we are aware of 32 case reports (DM 21, JDM 1, 2 overlap, PM 8), where the disease onset occurred during pregnancy. Most of these patients (16/32, 50%) presented in the 1st trimester, ten out of 32 (31%) presented in the 3rd trimester. It was the first pregnancy for 44% of them (14/32). The outcome is shown in Table 8.6.2. Six miscarriages and two neonatal deaths were observed with myositis onset during the 1st trimester. However, most of the 1st trimester foetal deaths were described before 1984. It is likely, with advances in the management of myositis and in obstetric practice, these figures might not reflect the current situation.

Onset of disease during puerperal period

There are 16 reported cases of new onset myositis during the puerperal period (ranging from 3 days to 4 months of the postpartum period). Seven of them followed the delivery of a healthy child, however, two babies were growth restricted, three had had a miscarriage, and two had stillbirths at 32 and 38 weeks respectively. This indicates a less favourable obstetric outcome; however the number of cases is too limited to draw conclusions.

In our case, the patient presented with myositis when she was 8 weeks pregnant. She was managed with an immunosuppressant compatible with pregnancy (see Chapter 3) and is afterwards followed up closely. Given her new diagnosis and the possible impact on her pregnancy outcome, this lady was closely followed up under the rheumatology, obstetric and respiratory teams. Multidisciplinary communication in this setting was extremely important to ensure that the patient received adequate treatment and no conflicting information regarding her immunosuppressive treatment. She required rituximab during pregnancy to manage her second flare at week 20 (given rituximab at week 22). Rituximab is a monoclonal antibody against CD20 positive B cells. In this

Table 8.6.2 Complications with onset of myositis during pregnancy in different trimesters

Category (n = 32)*	Total	Pregnancy complication
Third trimester	10	1 small-for-gestational-age
Second trimester	6	1 IUGR** 1 elective abortion (because of interstitial lung disease)
First trimester	16	6 abortions 2 neonatal deaths 4 premature deliveries 1 IUGR 1 emergency Caesarean section due to placenta praevia

*The n=32 figure is derived from a literature search; the most important of these references are shown in the Further reading list.
**IUGR= Intrauterine growth restriction.

case, it was necessary to administer rituximab during the 2nd trimester in order to manage her potentially life-threatening disease.

Case 3: Treatment of myositis during pregnancy

A 27-year-old pregnant (18 weeks, first pregnancy) white Caucasian female, who was previously diagnosed with anti-threonyl-tRNA (anti-PL 7) associated anti-synthetase syndrome, presented to the acute emergency department with a 2-day history of shortness of breath with proximal weakness and pedal oedema for 7 days. She had initially presented 8 years ago with DM and lung fibrosis [honeycombing and lower lobe ground glass opacities on high resolution computed tomography (HRCT) of the lungs; forced vital capacity (FVC) was 73% of the predicted and diffusion capacity (dLCO) was 68% of the predicted, but stable appearance over the last 8 years]. She did not have typical mechanic hands or pulmonary hypertension. Her CK was raised 1,800 IU/L; anti-PL 7 antibody was positive. She was taking azathioprine (125 mg daily) and prednisolone (5 mg daily). On admission, her respiratory rate was 32, pulse 98 beats per minute, blood pressure 110/78 mm Hg, and oxygen saturation was 92% on room air. She had no cough, fever, haemoptysis, sputum, or pleurisy. On clinical examination, she had marked pedal oedema, raised JVP, and course crackles throughout the lung field. However, her heart sounds were normal and clinically there was no ascites. Moreover, she also had increasing proximal muscle weakness. Her initial blood gas analysis suggested type 1 respiratory failure, bedside chest x-ray suggested gross pulmonary oedema, and electrocardiogram (ECG) suggested non-specific T wave inversion in lead V1–V6. She was commenced on high-flow oxygen along with IV frusemide. A further blood test showed a rising CK (5400 IU/L), slightly raised C-reactive protein, raised troponin T (450 ng/L, with no significant rise in a subsequent test), no proteinuria. Based on these findings, myocarditis with associated flare of anti-synthetase syndrome was suspected. An urgent echocardiogram confirmed depressed ventricular function. Subsequently she was given IV methylprednisolone (1 g for 3 days) followed by oral prednisolone 20 mg/day. She initially responded quite well to steroids and diuretics. Cardiology, intensive care unit, and the obstetrics team were also closely involved. Fortunately, at that point her pregnancy was viable. Unfortunately, her muscle weakness progressed over the next few days which subsequently affected her swallowing but not her respiratory muscles. At that point, intravenous immunoglobulin (IVIG) was given and azathioprine was switched to tacrolimus 2 mg bd. Subsequently, her condition was stabilized. She was maintained on prednisolone, tacrolimus, and monthly IVIG. Her condition remained stable throughout the rest of her pregnancy and she gave birth to a healthy baby. Table 8.6.3 summarize the investigations which need to be considered in myositis associated with pregnancies.

Case discussion

Current practice guidelines from the British Society for Rheumatology (BSR) recommend that azathioprine (<2 mg/kg/day), hydroxychloroquine (200–400 mg/day), and

Table 8.6.3 Investigations to consider in women with myositis associated with pregnancy

Routine blood test	1. FBC*—mild anaemia, and mild increase of white cell may be seen in pregnancy 2. ESR**—can be raised in pregnancy 3. CRP***—can be mildly raised in 2nd trimester of pregnancy 4. renal function test 5. liver function test—ALT^ and AST^^ can be raised not only in myositis, but also in pregnancy induced toxaemia 6. bone profile specially calcium
Urine test	urine for dipstick, routine microscopy, and myoglobin (to see any evidence of rhabdomyolysis)
Muscle enzymes	CK^^^ Aldolase LDH~
Auto-antibodies	ANA‡ anti-dsDNA ENA‡‡‡ muscle-specific antibodies anti-phospholipid antibodies
Further test and imaging	EMG† MRI of muscle, but gadolinium enhanced MRI should not be done due to possible adverse effects on child outcome (20)
Biopsy	Muscle and skin biopsy

*FBC = Full blood count, ** ESR= Erythrocyte sedimentation rate, ***CRP= C - reactive protein, ^ALT= Alanine transferase, ^^AST= Aspartate transferase, ^^^CK=Creatine kinase, ~ LDH= Lactate dehydrogenase, ‡ANA= Anti- nuclear antibody, ‡‡anti-dsDNA= anti-double stranded DNA, ‡‡‡ ENA= Extractable nuclear antigen, †EMG= Electromyography.

ciclosporin/tacrolimus (with close monitoring of maternal blood pressure, renal function, blood glucose, and drug level) are safe during pregnancy. So, these medications should be continued when patients become pregnant to ensure better disease control. However, mycophenolate mofetil (should be stopped 6 weeks in advance) and methotrexate (should be stopped 3 months in advance) are not recommended (see Chapter 3.1).

A caveat with the use of steroids is that doses above 20 mg are associated with a significant increase in complications such as gestational diabetes, hypertension, infections, and premature ruptures of membranes, if used for long periods. However, existing reported cases have not found any incremental risk of pregnancy losses. IVIG has been used successfully and may be an effective alternative to high-dose corticosteroids, although small numbers of patients have been treated with IVIG.

The BSR recommends that rituximab (RTX) should not be given for at least 6 months prior to pregnancy (16). Limited evidence, however, has not shown RTX to be teratogenic and only 2nd-/3rd-trimester exposure is associated with neonatal B

```
┌─────────────────────────────────────────────────────────────┐
│                        In acute flare:                       │
│  1st line: Prednisolone with or without intravenous           │
│             methylprednisolone.                               │
│  2nd line:  Intravenous immunoglobulin (IVIG) (when can't     │
│  taper off or tolerate steroid, or no response to steroid).   │
└─────────────────────────────────────────────────────────────┘
                            ▼
┌─────────────────────────────────────────────────────────────┐
│   Maintenance-first line steroid-sparing immunosuppressant    │
│                           agent:                              │
│     Consider dose increment/add/switch (whichever appropriate)│
│     Azathioprine (AZA), Ciclosporin (CSA), Tacrolimus (TAC).  │
│  Adjuvant: Hydroxychloroquine for skin manifestations of      │
│  dermatomyositis.                                             │
└─────────────────────────────────────────────────────────────┘
                            ▼
┌─────────────────────────────────────────────────────────────┐
│                       Resistant case:                         │
│   Second line: Consider combination of AZA with CSA/TAC.      │
│   Third line: Consider rituximab (RTX)/cyclophosphamide (RTX  │
│   probably safe in first trimester; in any other cases should │
│   only be consider in severe or life-/organ-threatening       │
│   maternal disease)                                           │
└─────────────────────────────────────────────────────────────┘
```

Figure 8.6.1 Treatment strategies in pregnancy associated myositis

cell depletion. Therefore, unintentional RTX exposure early in the 1st trimester is unlikely to be harmful (17). There are a few reported cases where RTX has been used in myositis who presented during pregnancy (18, 19). Cyclophosphamide has also been used, but in only a few cases (8). As per BSR guideline it should only be considered in pregnancy if a life-/organ-threatening condition is present.

Based on current practice and existing data the treatment strategy outlined in Figure 8.6.1 can be adopted.

Treatment options during breastfeeding

Azathioprine, hydroxychloroquine, prednisone, ciclosporin, tacrolimus, and IVIG have been recommended to be continued during breastfeeding, however the level of evidence is poor (see Chapter 3.1). There are no reliable data about the use of RTX.

Summary

Due to the paucity of data concerning pregnancy in myositis patients it is hard to draw firm conclusions. Fertility seems to be unaffected. Active disease and new onset of disease during the 1st trimester of pregnancy seem likely to increase the risk of adverse foetal outcome. However, optimizing myositis therapy along with better obstetric care does seem to have resulted in better outcome recently.

None the less, caution needs to be exercised and patients should be fully educated about the increased risk as active disease and early onset of myositis during pregnancy are associated with poor foetal outcome. Maternal health can also be a significant issue, especially due to the exposure to excessive prednisolone. There is limited evidence about the effectiveness of the many treatment modalities used in active disease, but IVIG is an alternative option to steroids. Among the conventional treatments, azathioprine, hydroxychloroquine, ciclosporin, and tacrolimus have been recommended as safe.

Key messages

- Inflammatory myositis can first present during pregnancies and puerperal periods.
- Active myositis and earlier onset (1st trimester) of myositis during pregnancy may be associated with poor foetal outcome.
- Active disease may increase the risk of foetal death, premature birth, and IUGR.
- The outcome is favourable if the disease is in remission.
- Steroid can increase risk of gestational diabetes, hypertension, and premature rupture of membranes.
- IVIG may be an option to treat active disease during pregnancy.
- Azathioprine (<2 mg/kg/day), hydroxychloroquine, ciclosporin, and tacrolimus are compatible with pregnancy and can be continued during breastfeeding.

Further reading

1. Silva CA, Sultan SM, Isenberg DA. Pregnancy outcome in adult-onset idiopathic inflammatory myopathy. *Rheumatology*. 2003;42:1168–72.
2. Chopra S, Suri V, MD; Rashmi R, et al. Autoimmune inflammatory myopathy in pregnancy. *Medscape J Med*. 2008;10:17.
3. King CR, Chow S. Dermatomyositis and pregnancy. *Obstet Gynecol*. 1985;66:589–92.
4. Gutierrez G, Dagnino R, Mintz G. Polymyositis/dermatomyositis and pregnancy. *Arthritis Rheum*. 1984;27:291–4.
5. Al-Adnani M, Kiho L, Scheimberg I. Recurrent placental massive perivillous fibrin deposition associated with polymyositis: A case report and review of the literature. *Pediatr Dev Pathol*. 2010;11(3):226–9.
6. Hung NA, Jackson C, Nicholson, et al. Pregnancy-related polymyositis and massive perivillous fibrin deposit in the placenta: Are they pathologically related? *Arthritis Rheum*. 2006;55(1):154–6.

7. Takei R, Suzuki S, Kijima K, et al. First presentation of polymyositis postpartum following intrauterine fetal death. *Arch Gynecol Obstet.* 2000;47(8):264.

8. Steiner I, Averbuch-Heller L, Abramsky O, et al. Postpartum idiopathic polymyositis. *Lancet.* 1992;339:256.

9. Satoh M, Ajmani AK, Hirakata M, et al. Onset of myositis with antibodies to threonyl-tRNA synthey tase during pregnancy. *J Rheumatol.* 1994;21:1564–6

10. Kupferminc M, Rimon E, Many A, et al. Low molecular weight heparin versus no treatment in women with previous severe pregnancy complications and placental findings without thrombophilia. *Blood Coagul Fibrinolysis.* 2011;22:123–6.

11. Kolstad KD, Fiorentino D, Li S, et al. Pregnancy outcomes in adult patients with dermatomyositis and polymyositis. *Semin Arthritis Rheum.* 2017;47:865–9.

12. Akalin T, Akkaya H, Büke B, et al. A case of new-onset dermatomyositis in the second trimester of pregnancy: A case report and review of the literature. *Case Rep Obstet Gynecol.* 2016: [Published online 2016, 10 Jul. doi: 10.1155/2016/6430156.

13. Missumi LS, Souza FHC, Andrade JQ, et al. Pregnancy outcomes in dermatomyositis and polymyositis patients. *Revista Brasileira de Reumatologia.* 2015;55:95–102.

14. Di Martino SJ. Myositis and Pregnancy. In: Sammaritano LR, Bermas BL. *Contraception and pregnancy in patients with rheumatic disease.* New York: Springer. 2014;185–97. See: https://link.springer.com/book/10.1007%2F978-1-4939-0673-4.

15. Miller FW, Chen W, O'Hanlon TP, et al. Genome-wide association study identifies HLA 8.1 ancestral haplotype alleles as major genetic risk factors for myositis phenotypes. *Genes Immun.* 2015;16:470–80.

16. Flint J, Panchal S, Hurrell A, et al. BSR and BHPR guideline on prescribing drugs in pregnancy and breastfeeding: Standard and biologic disease modifying anti-rheumatic drugs and corticosteroids. *Rheumatology.* 2016;55(9):1693–7.

17. Chakravarty EF, Murray ER, Kelman A, et al. Pregnancy outcomes after maternal exposure to rituximab. *Blood.* 2011;117:1499–506.

18. Mehta P, Dorsey-Campbell R, Dassan P, et al. Difficult case: Rituximab in anti-SRP antibody myositis in pregnancy. *Pract Neurol.* 2019;19(5):444–6.

19. Etomi O, Mehta P, Nelson-Piercy C, et al. Inflammatory myositis in pregnancy. The value of early diagnosis and aggressive treatment: A case series. *Pregnancy Hypertension.* 2018;13(1):146.

20. Ray JG, Vermeulen MJ, Bharatha A, et al. Association between MRI exposure during pregnancy and fetal and childhood outcomes. *JAMA.* 2016;316:952–61.

8.7

Ankylosing spondylitis in pregnancy

Monika Østensen

Background

Ankylosing spondylitis (AS) typically affects individuals in the 3rd decade of life and is in its radiographic form predominant in men with a male to female ratio of 2:1 whereas the non-radiographic form has an equal gender distribution. Disease expression is somewhat different in the genders. Men develop more severe radiological changes of the spine; women suffer more widespread axial and peripheral pain and greater functional impairment (1).

Several studies have investigated the effect of pregnancy on the disease course and symptom severity of axial spondyloarthritis (axSpA), previously called ankylosing spondylitis. In contrast to rheumatoid arthritis pregnancy does not improve the symptoms of AS. Compared to the non-pregnant state, disease activity is mostly not substantially altered during pregnancy, and about 80% of AS women have active disease (defined as ankylosing spondylitis disease activity score (ASDAS)-C-reactive protein (CRP)>2.1) at some stage of pregnancy. A flare is commonly seen in the 2nd trimester when about 45% of patients experience aggravation of disease and intensified pain at inflammation sites (2). Nocturnal pain disturbing sleep, morning stiffness lasting for hours, and occasionally sudden swelling of a peripheral joint or anterior uveitis accompany the flare. Increased disease activity is most often accompanied by elevated CRP levels. Need for anti-inflammatory drugs increases during a flare and is present in about 70% of the patients (3). The symptoms do not respond to corticosteroids, even to doses exceeding 30 mg/day. Alleviation of inflammation is often seen in the 3rd trimester with a reduction of biochemical inflammation markers; however, physical functioning may be worst at this time due to the increasing weight of the foetus.

In patients studied during multiple pregnancies, intensity of disease symptoms varied from one pregnancy to the other, and no uniform pattern regarding improvement or aggravation emerged. However, complete remission of symptoms never occurred in any patient with pure spinal disease (4).

Pregnancy outcome correlates with disease severity. In women with well-controlled axSpA and no comorbidities the disease has no harmful effect on the course of pregnancy or on foetal wellbeing. Patients who are continued on effective therapy and remain on stable low disease activity have pregnancies concluding at term with the delivery of live, healthy children of normal birth weight (5). The rate of miscarriage is within the limits for healthy women. Premature delivery and small-for-gestational-age infants are increased in patients with very active disease or with comorbidities (6).

Maternal disease activity postpartum: in previous retrospective studies, 40–60% of patients with AS reported aggravation of symptoms 4–12 weeks after delivery. Episodes of acute peripheral arthritis or anterior uveitis occurred 1.5–3 times more often postpartum than during pregnancy (2). Clinical signs were accompanied by elevations of CRP. The postpartum flare was unrelated to resumption of menstruation or lactation. One study found the flare correlated to active disease at conception, but unrelated to disease activity during pregnancy. Of note, many of these patients had received no treatment during pregnancy or postpartum or were undertreated. In recent prospective studies, a postpartum flare was less frequent, but most patients had restarted a synthetic or biological disease-modifying drug (DMARD) within 6 months after delivery (5). Disease activity returned as a rule to the pre-pregnancy pattern during the year following delivery.

Case 1: Vaginal delivery or Caesarean section in a patient with axSpA?

A 29-year-old woman was diagnosed with axSpA 4 years ago. At the time of diagnosis, the patient was complaining of symptoms suggestive of sacroiliac and lumbar spine involvement. Radiographs did show inflammatory lesions at both sites. No peripheral joints have been involved but enthesitis at the heel has occurred.

In the first year after diagnosis the patient had relief of pain and stiffness by therapy with diclofenac, later sulfasalazine (SZ) was added because of intensifying symptoms and additional enthesitis at both heels. However, the effect was not optimal and SZ was stopped. During the last year the patient has been treated with etanercept bi-weekly with good control of disease symptoms. The patient is now pregnant with her first child. Her rheumatologist has advised her to continue etanercept at the same dose throughout pregnancy. Except for short periods of back pain and enthesitis, no aggravation has occurred during pregnancy. The patient is currently 35 weeks pregnant and asks whether she needs to have a Caesarean section or whether she can deliver vaginally. She is concerned that the inflammation in her sacroiliac joints could render parturition difficult. She has discussed this with her obstetrician who felt uncertain about the issue.

Case discussion

The rate of Caesarean section has been found to be twice to three times as high in women with AS compared to healthy pregnant women (4). When separating emergency from elective Caesarean section surgical delivery is most often not significantly increased in women with AS. In the absence of foetal problems or pregnancy-related complications elective Caesarean section may depend on disease severity, and the preference of the patient or the obstetrician.

It also occurs that the anaesthesiologist is hesitant to administer an epidural anaesthesic to a woman with AS, because she/he fears problems in case there should be ankylosis of the spine. The placement of the epidural catheter could be difficult or at presence of calcifications in the ligamentum dorsi the anaesthetic agent may not spread optimally. These concerns can be overcome by performing an x-ray of the lumbar spine before a planned pregnancy and by ultrasound-guided central nerve block at parturition.

Inflammation or ankylosis of the sacroiliac joints is not a mechanical hindrance for the progression of parturition. Also, hip disease or total hip replacement does not preclude normal delivery though the presence of these complications is rare. Ankylosis of the spine is much less frequent in women with AS than in men and occurs only after decades of active inflammation. Most women with AS can therefore have a vaginal delivery.

Case 2: Flare in a patient with spondyloarthropathy in the 2nd trimester

A 31-year-old woman with axSpA diagnosed at the age of 23, bilateral sacroiliitis confirmed by magnetic resonance (MR) and later on by radiographs. Initial treatment with diclofenac and SZ, but after 2 years change to adalimumab with good effect.

The patient became pregnant and decided to discontinue adalimumab at week 5 of gestation. Four weeks later she experienced arthritis in her left knee and increasing pain in the sacroiliac joints. She tried diclofenac 50 mg × 3/day with some relief, but her arthritis persisted. An intraarticular corticosteroid injection was given into the left knee and both sacroiliac joints with temporary effect. At gestational week 18 she suffered a severe aggravation with intensive back pain during the night and long-lasting morning stiffness. She also experienced intense pain at enthesitis sites and complained of lack of energy. She could not continue her work as a teacher. Peroral prednisone 40 mg/day improved knee joint arthritis but not the spinal symptoms. Her general practitioner asked the rheumatologist whether he should restart adalimumab at week 20 or change to certolizumab. He also wanted to know whether therapy should be given throughout pregnancy.

Case discussion

This case highlights several problems which may occur in pregnant women with AS. The first is the discontinuation of adalimumab in the 1st trimester. Stop of an effective immunosuppressive therapy often results in a flare (7). In the patient described, not only the spinal symptoms relapsed but she also developed de novo arthritis in a peripheral joint. Symptoms did not respond to non-steroidal anti-inflammatory drugs (NSAIDs), nor did they abate when intra-articular and peroral prednisone were given. The resistance of axSpA to corticosteroids is known: 20 mg of prednisone is without effect and doses of ≥50 mg have moderate effect. Since women with AS frequently have active arthritis at some stage of pregnancy, immunosuppressive therapy should not be stopped but continued throughout pregnancy. In women who have low or no disease activity a dose reduction of the tumour necrosis factor (TNF) inhibitor can be tried under close monitoring.

The question whether the type of TNF inhibitor should be changed during pregnancy can be debated. Some specialists would argue that a switch of biologic in a patient who is well-established and in remission on any anti-TNF therapy should be avoided, whereas others would prefer to switch a patient to an anti-TNF therapy with minimal placental transfer. There is currently no international consensus, and any treatment choice should therefore be made together with the patient on an individual basis.

A complete monoclonal antibody such as adalimumab given throughout pregnancy is actively transported through the placenta by the foetal Fc-receptor and reaches a high concentration in the foetus in the 3rd trimester with the level in cord blood exceeding maternal levels at birth. Due to the prolonged half-life of antibodies in the newborn, live vaccines should not be given during the first 6 months to children exposed in the 2nd or 3rd trimester to biologics.

Pegylated certolizumab which is an Fc-free anti-TNF drug, has no active transplacental transport and is not or minimally detected in cord blood. The advantage of restarting adalimumab during pregnancy would be the knowledge that it has kept the patient in remission before conception. Whether the patient will respond in the same way to certolizumab is not known. However, certolizumab has no or minimal placental transfer. Any decision to switch anti-tumour necrosis factor (anti-TNF) therapy highlights the importance of pregnancy counselling, as a switch ideally should be followed by a period of observation to ensure that the patient remains in remission under the alternatively established treatment.

For the patient who has active arthritis in one or a limited number of joints, intra-articular steroid injection(s) can be useful. In patients with AS, analgesics such as acetaminophen or low-dose corticosteroids are frequently insufficient in controlling the often-intense nocturnal pain and the long-lasting morning stiffness of the spine. NSAIDs or non-selective and selective cyclooxygenase (COX) inhibitors are more effective in this respect. NSAID can be used in the first half of gestation since there is no indication that salicylates, phenylbutazone, indomethacin, fenoprofen, ibuprofen, ketoprofen, naproxen, diclofenac, mefenamic acid, and piroxicam do harm the developing foetus (see Chapter 3.1). At present, we do not know whether this is also true for the so-called selective COX2 inhibitors celecoxib and etoricoxib. They should therefore be stopped at the start of pregnancy. Since NSAIDs may have dose-dependent adverse effects on the foetus when given in full anti-inflammatory dose one should target to administer the smallest effective dose. NSAIDs can constrict the prostaglandin-dependent opening of the ductus arteriosus which bypasses the lung in foetal life and impair renal function of the foetus. Side effects can be avoided when NSAIDs are withdrawn 10–8 weeks before delivery or the development of side effects in the foetus is monitored by repeated ultrasonography. Both constriction of the ductus arteriosus and reduced renal function resolve within 1–5 days after withdrawal of the drug. In the 2nd and early-3rd trimester only NSAIDs with a short or medium half-life should be administered.

Key messages

- The typical pattern of AS is active disease during the 1st and early-2nd trimester, frequently accompanied by a mid-gestational flare around week 20.
- Medication controlling AS effectively before conception should be continued during pregnancy but follow the recommendations given for gestational use of the drug class.
- Pregnancy outcome is within the rates for healthy women except in patients with very active disease or with comorbidities.
- Sacroiliitis and spinal inflammation are no indications for surgical delivery, though structural changes in the lumbar spine may render epidural anaesthesia difficult.

Further reading

1. Tournadre A, Pereira B, Lhoste A, Dubost JJ, Ristori JM, Claudepierre P, Dougados M, Soubrier M. Differences between women and men with recent-onset axial spondyloarthritis: Results from a prospective multicenter French cohort. *Arthritis Care Res* (Hoboken). 2013;65(9):1482–9.
2. Østensen M, Østensen H. Ankylosing spondylitis—the female aspect. *J Rheumatol.* 1998;25:120–4.
3. Østensen M, Fuhrer L, Renateu R, Seitz M, Villiger PM. A prospective study of pregnant patients with rheumatoid arthritis and ankylosing spondylitis using validated clinical instruments. *Ann Rheum Dis.* 2004;63:1212–17.
4. Østensen M, Dolhain R, Ruiz-Irastorza G. Obstetrics and Pregnancy. In: *Oxford Textbook of Rheumatology* 4e. Eds. Richard A. Watts, Philip G. Conaghan, Christopher Denton, Helen Foster, John Isaacs, Ulf Müller-Ladner. Oxford: Oxford University Press, 2018.
5. Ursin K, Lydersen S, Skomsvoll JF, Wallenius M. Disease activity during and after pregnancy in women with axial spondyloarthritis: A prospective multicentre study. *Rheumatology* (Oxford). 2018;57(6):1064–71.
6. Jakobsson GL, Stephansson O, Askling J, Jacobsson LT. Pregnancy outcomes in patients with ankylosing spondylitis: A nationwide register study. *Ann Rheum Dis.* 2016;75(10):1838–42.
7. van den Brandt S, Zbinden A, Baeten D, Villiger PM, Østensen M, Förger F. Risk factors for flare and treatment of disease flares during pregnancy in RA and SpA patients. *Arthritis Res Ther.* 2017;19(1):64.

Summary table for medication use during pregnancy

Medication name	Teratogenicity	Use in pregnancy	Lactation	Comments
Conventional DMARDs				
Azathioprine	none identified	compatible	compatible	safe to use all trimesters
Cyclophosphamide	possible teratogen	life- or organ-threatening disease	avoid	2nd & 3rd trimester use for life- or organ-threatening disease
Ciclosporin	none identified	compatible	compatible	safe to use all trimesters
Hydroxychloroquine	none identified	compatible	compatible	may reduce lupus flares, may reduce CHB in SSA+ women, safe to use in all trimesters
Leflunomide	suspected teratogen	avoid	avoid	requires cholestyramine washout
Methotrexate	known teratogen	avoid	controversial	rate of birth defects ~10%
Mycophenolate mofetil	known teratogen	avoid	avoid	discontinue 1–3 months prior to pregnancy
Prednisone	minimal increased risk of cleft palate	compatible	compatible	use lowest dose possible; rapid onset of action for acute disease flares
Sulfasalazine	none identified	compatible	compatible	safe to use all trimesters
Tacrolimus	none identified	compatible	compatible	safe to use all trimesters
Biological DMARDs				
Abatacept	unknown	unknown	compatible	use if no other drug controls moderate to severe disease

Adalimumab	none identified	compatible	compatible	transplacental transfer in later pregnancy
Anakinra	unknown	unknown	compatible	use if no other drug controls moderate to severe disease
Belimumab	unknown	unknown	compatible	use if no other drug controls moderate to severe disease
Canakinumab	unknown	unknown	compatible	use if no other drug controls moderate to severe disease
Certolizumab	none identified	compatible	compatible	minimal transplacental transfer
Etanercept	none identified	compatible	compatible	minimal transplacental transfer
Golimumab	none identified	compatible	compatible	transplacental transfer in later pregnancy
Infliximab	none identified	compatible	compatible	transplacental transfer in later pregnancy
Rituximab	none identified	Life- or organ-threatening disease	compatible	use for life- or organ-threatening disease
Tocilizumab	unknown	unknown	compatible	use if no other drug controls moderate to severe disease
Other				
Warfarin	known teratogen	switch to heparin	compatible	
ACE inhibitors	known teratogen	Life- or organ-threatening disease	compatible, monitor infant BP	1st trimester exposure birth defects (debated), 2nd & 3rd trimester foetotoxic

Key: ACE inhibitors – angiotensin converting enzyme inhibitors; DMARD – disease-modifying antirheumatic drug.

Index

Note: Tables, figures and boxes are indicated by *t*, *f* and *b* following the page number